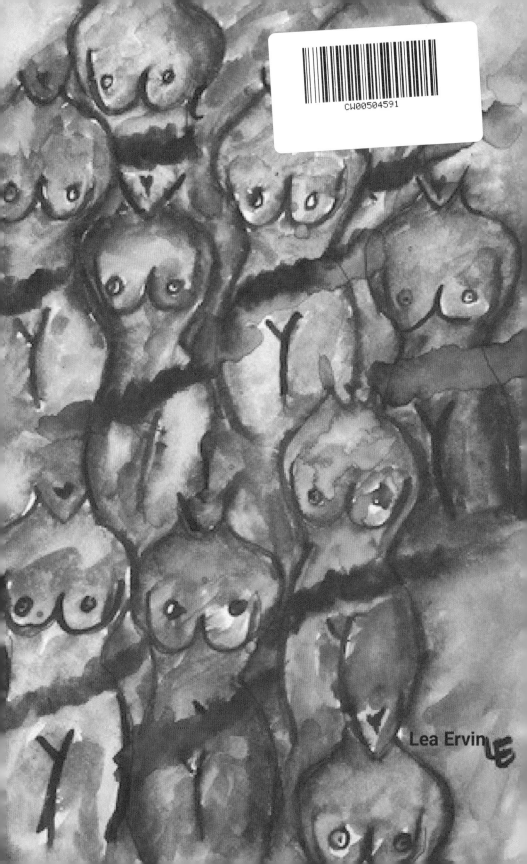

Lea Ervin

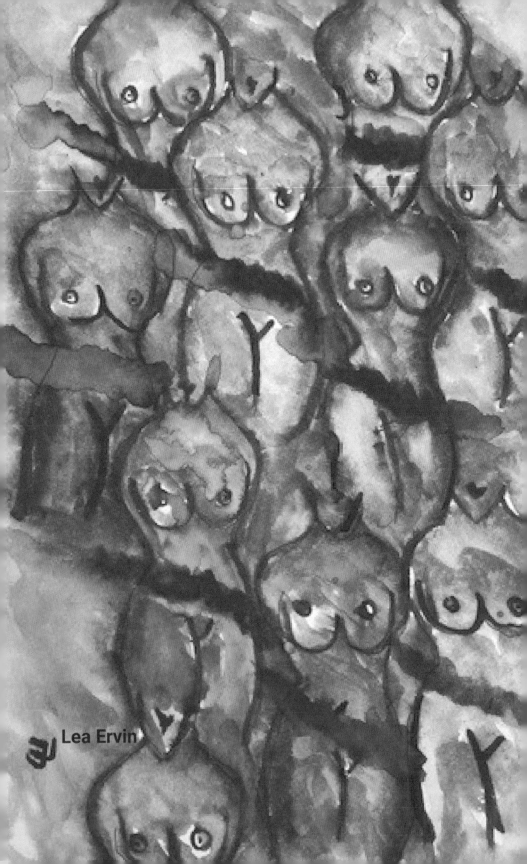

Lea Ervin

All events, beliefs and characters portrayed are based on the individual author's recollection and interpretation of past events and understanding of their medical condition. Each poem has been reviewed by the poet, and all comments have been unedited so there may be spelling or grammar errors present.

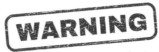

Content warning: discussion may include but not limited to topics such as miscarriage, medical trauma, infertility, depression and gaslighting.

All proceeds from the sale of '1-IN-10 Poetry' will directly support current and future Satirev projects, including but not limited to Project 514 415, In which all authors and artists have given permission to Project 514 415 to publish their works to support Project 514 415 Mission and raise funds for future projects.

Satirev Publishing
London, UK

First edition 2024

British Library Cataloguing in Publication Data
A catalogue record for this book is available from the British Library

ISBN: 978-1-0687164-0-9 (Hardback)
ISBN: 978-1-0687164-1-6 (Paperback)
ISBN: 978-1-0687164-2-3 (EBook)

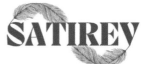

In loving memory of

Terrence Conway

Terrence was a caring husband, father, and grandfather who played a crucial role in supporting his daughter, Candice, throughout her struggle with endometriosis and her advocacy efforts in Scotland.

Terrence Conway, a artist from Scotland, supported Project 514 415 and contributed two artworks to Project 514 415.

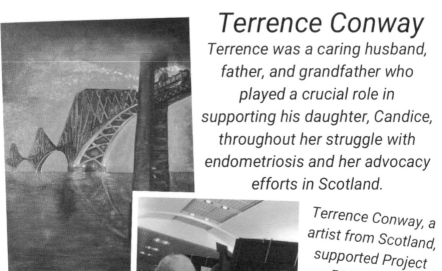

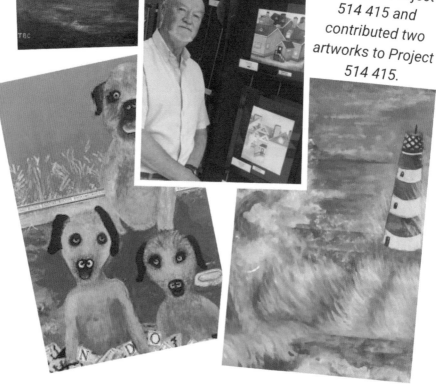

Artists Disclaimer

All art work is owned by each individual artist, in which they have given Project 514 415 permission to publish their work showcasing their experiences with endometriosis. Please contact the artist directly for sales or commissions.

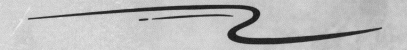

Artist contact details

Lea Ervin...@grungetta82

Morten Naess..www.moga-art.com

Susanne Jenssen..@artofsusie

Alice Brunello Luise....................................@alicebrunelloluise_ph

Iness Rychlik..www.inessrychlik.com

Clare Gregory..@_.clareellen

Gazelle Pezeshkmehr.......................................www.moga-art.com

Terrence Conway...@endowarriorswl

Charlotte Montgomery..........charlottemontygomery@gmail.com

Leonie Thoby..@leonieillustrations

Alysia J. Dagrosa...@TantieLys

Emma Boittiaux...@emmaboittiaux

Savannah Dasilva..@sdasilva_art

Please note that a variety of artistic mediums have been used by each individual artist including but not limited to: textiles, oil painting, graphic design, collage, photography and AI technology.

Artists Disclaimer

All art work used during our awareness campaign is owned by each individual artist, in which they have given Project 514 415 permission to publish their work showcasing their experiences with endometriosis, to raise awareness for endometriosis symptoms. Please contact the artist directly for sales or commissions.

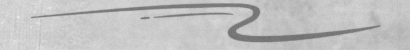

Artist contact details

Arti Shah ....@artiphotography

Abigail Fraser...@endowarriorabi

Andrea Neph...@momminwithendo

Anonymous...@unmaskedendo

Alexandra Peters ....@endoandme2023

Charlotte Montgomery...........charlottemontygomery@gmail.com

Mike Baker (Endo dad)...@endodad76

Marguerita Cruz-Urbanc.......................................@mmargueritacu

Macarena Valenzuela...@poderosautera

Natalie Murtagh...@nat.niamh.tattoos

Zoe Almendarez...Anonymous

Lea Ervin..@grungetta82

Please note that a variety of artistic mediums have been used by each individual artist including but not limited to: textiles, oil painting, graphic design, collage, photography and AI technology.

Acknowledgments

I never anticipated the challenges that would come with writing and editing a collaborative poetry book. None of this would have been achievable without the invaluable support and opinions of Chelsea, Aimee, Jessie and Candice. I am deeply grateful that our chance encounter united us under my vision of debunking misconceptions, supporting the endometriosis community and creating a better future for the next generation of people living with endometriosis. Chelsea's & Aimee's unwavering dedication has been instrumental in supporting both Project 514 415 and the editing process, while also offering a safe space to vent and share a joke.

We express our gratitude for Jessie's poetry workshop, where she inspired the creation of several poems. Organizing five poetry sessions for individuals with endometriosis, Jessie encouraged participants to express the impacts of endometriosis through poetry. Many attendees appreciated the workshops and the opportunity to explore their personal experiences.

I am deeply thankful to everyone who shared their personal experiences with endometriosis and took part in our survey. The artistic and literary submissions have been truly powerful, meaningful, and distinctive. I am enthusiastic about expanding

Project 514 415 to highlight the diverse experiences of endometriosis. The dream one day is to organize a comprehensive exhibition showcasing these experiences, offering a platform for sharing stories and providing essential resources and education to both the endometriosis community and wider public.

A heartfelt thank you goes out to all the artists and poets who participated in creating the 1-in-10 poetry book. Your combined efforts have given this collection a voice, shedding light on the true experiences of endometriosis.

I want to express my gratitude to our wonderful sponsors who generously contributed to project 514 415. Their vital support has allowed us to finish the '1-IN-10 Poetry' book in addition to other projects.

A special thank you to our ambassadors; Kirstin, Eman, Ashlee, Kristen and Amelie for their valuable contributions to Project 514 415. We are truly grateful for all your efforts and look forward to collaborating on upcoming projects.

Without Yasmin, Project 514 415 wouldn't exist. After two years of brainstorming Yasmin encouraged me to kickstart Project 514 415. Thank you for believing in me and my vision.

Lastly, I would like to thank my mother for devoting her evenings helping me to shortlist over 100 poems.

Contents

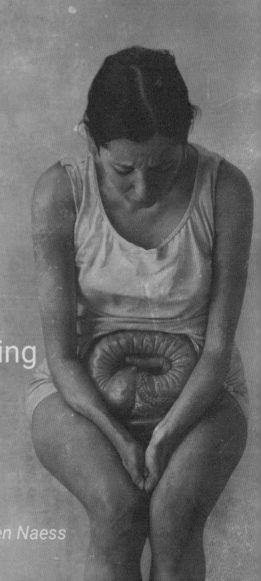

Introduction

Endometriosis

Gas Lighting

Flare up

Surgery

Despair

Support

Inspired

Poetry Journaling

The Results

They Said

Artist: Morten Naess

Endometriosis is a systemic, inflammatory disease characterised by the presence of endometrium-like tissue found outside the uterine cavity.

(Kennedy S. et al., 2005; Klemmt et al., 2018; Saunders et al 2021, International working group of AAGL, ESGE, ESHRE and WES et al 2021)

Campaign initiated by Rey (@reythewarrior)

"Microsurgical principles are of paramount importance to improve patient outcomes in surgeries. These tenets should be uniformly applied in all surgical procedures. As surgeons who perform minimally invasive surgeries, they must revisit these principles and advocate for their training and universal implementation. Nonadherence to microsurgical principles can result in detrimental surgical outcomes, including adhesions, parasitic myomas, port site metastasis, peritonitis, and compromised ovarian reserve."

Nezhat C, McGrail K, Hincapie M. Revisiting microsurgical principles for the minimally invasive surgeon. Fertil Steril. 2023 Jan;119(1):151-152. doi: 10.1016/j.fertnstert.2022.10.008. Epub 2022 Nov 19. PMID: 36414478.

In adolescence, the most common cause of secondary dysmenorrhea is endometriosis.

Dixon S, Vincent K, Hirst J, Hippisley-Cox J. Incidence of menstrual symptoms suggestive of possible endometriosis in adolescents: and variance in these by ethnicity and socio-economic status. Br J Gen Pract. 2024 Jun 20;74(suppl 1):bjgp24x737685.

Delays in the diagnosis of endometriosis are common and are associated with a worsened quality of life and greater medical costs

Darba J, Marsa A. Economic Implications of Endometriosis: A Review. Pharmacoeconomics. 2022 Nov 8.

What does 'Project 514 415' mean?

$$5 = E$$
$$14 = N$$
$$4 = D$$
$$15 = O$$

Project ENDO

Project 514 415

Project 514 415 was founded following my horrific experiences with endometriosis, like most I was heavily gaslit by medical professionals who treated me with medical bias and sexism. It took 20 years of self-managing blackouts, burning up, extreme rib & pelvic pain, throwing up, and fatigue, until my health and quality of life dramatically deteriorated, leaving me unable to manage my previous symptoms alongside my new symptoms of: blood in my stools, heart palpations, shortness of breath, night sweats, bilateral sciatica, stabbing pain in the shoulder and weight loss. Being completely dismissed by my GP and A&E as imagined pain over a clinically insignificant cyst which I have been told about and having anxiety/depression. Turning to the private sector for a second opinion, resulted in a bittersweet moment of finally having a diagnosis and rational explanation for my symptoms. However, being told I'd require IVF if I ever wanted a family in addition to a surgery that could result in a stoma from the damage that endometriosis has done to my organs was unexpected and overwhelming.

I left the consultation alone, bewildered and as though my envisioned future has just died in front of me. I spent hours wandering the eerily empty streets of London (COVID lockdown) trying to make sense of everything, plan for surgery and working out how I can take control of my future, until I ended up bursting into tears outside of a 'Joe & the Juice'. As I calmed down, I started to wonder how many other people have been through a similar experience, I never wanted anyone to feel as I felt in this moment, or for them to suffer unnecessarily due to their medical symptoms being dismissed due to misconceptions and medical bias.

Wanting to make an impactful difference to break this cycle and empower the endometriosis community with informed choices before it is too late. Project 514 415 was born with the mission to debunk misconceptions and to share the TRUE lived experience of endometriosis, banishing the old wives tale that further spread misinformation to both the medical profession and the public.

In the last four years, Project 514 415 has steadily developed, achieving the following milestones with the backing of the endometriosis community and our ambassadors:

- Launched a 2024 endometriosis campaign featuring artworks created by the endometriosis community, coupled with informative facts about the condition.
- Distributed thousands of endometriosis symptom postcards within the community.
- Held our first Art exhibition in Norway, hosted by Kristiansund Kunsthall contemporary Art gallery.

1-in-10 Poetry

Welcome to the 1-in-10 poetry book created and illustrated by the endometriosis community. This book showcases:

- 64 contributors
- 67 poems
- 28 artworks
- 166 voices from the lived experiences of an endometriosis survey
- 100 direct comments from individuals living with endometriosis

Organised into 10 chapters, 6 of which delve into themes significant to the endometriosis community, featuring 9 poems and an artwork reflecting on each theme. The remaining 4 chapters highlight our previous projects completed in the last 2 years.

Inspiration: Featuring 13 poems inspired by our 2024 endometriosis campaign, and selected by the artists.

Poetry Journaling: Offering 10 creative exercises to inspire your own poem writing.

The Results: Presenting the outcomes of our survey shedding light on current experiences affecting the endometriosis community.

They Said: Presenting 100 selected comments from the endometriosis community, sharing advice and recounting interactions with medical professionals.

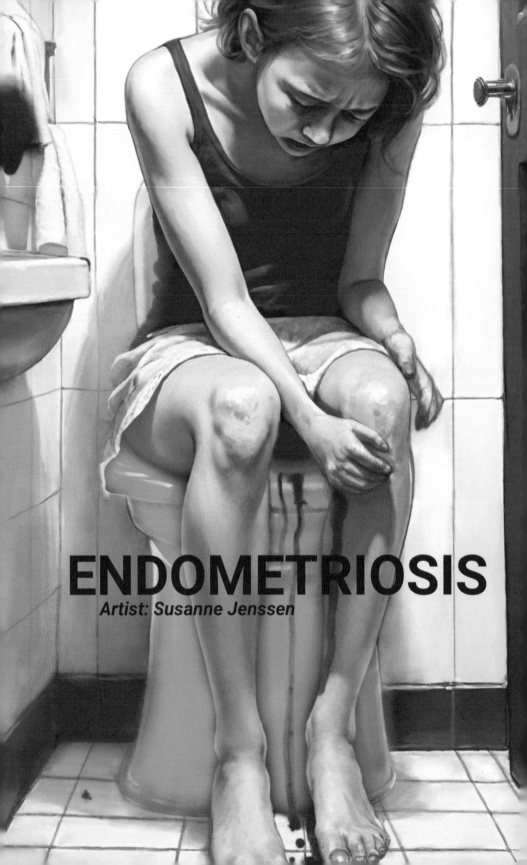

ENDOMETRIOSIS
Artist: Susanne Jenssen

Could you?

Could you cope?
Could you do it every day?
Awake with pain that stays all day.

Could you work?
Could you stay for a day?
Defeat the nausea as you slay the day.

Could you commute?
Could you stand all the way?
Whilst a dizzy spell sways you away.

Could you sleep?
Could you sleep the day away?
As barbed wire wraps your thigh.

By Aimee Gill

(Inspired by a short story submitted to project 514 415)

Endohood

My childhood dreams are lost at sea.
My hopes turned to fears that shouldn't be.

Gifted with more than a scar or three.
I stand frightened as can be.

The reflection of my past I wish to unseen.
The struggles of endohood that nearly destroyed me.

By Verity Kerr -Morrall

(Inspired by a short story submitted to project 514 415)

Endometriosis

Endometriosis is a condition that is no joke,
You are forced into a world not knowing how to cope.
Realising there is no cure makes your heart ache,
And leaves you wondering if you're in a nightmare or if you're awake.
The pain that comes is hard to explain,
The burning, the shocks, the shooting, the PAIN!

Losing your former self is hard,
And having operation after operation is so incredibly sad.
The isolation, being bed bound and struggling with life,
While watching others live their 'best life'.
The loss of organs and potential dreams,
Watching others have what you want and you trying not to be mean.

Smiling automatically to hide those flowing tears,
Feeling helpless and lost and full of so many fears.
Until one day, you find that place where you belong,
And find your community where for you, others are strong.
When others are at a loss of what to say,
And you find this condition has brought you to your knees to pray.

To pray for a cure and this you know for sure, That you would not be here without your support and family.

So, let's all be in this as one,
And really try to give it everything and some.
So that we come out, out on top,
Because you must know, that we will NEVER stop.

Even if it means we fight the fight,
We warriors do have all of the might!
So, Endometriosis, we are telling you,
We are coming, we are coming for YOU!

By Prabhjot Kaur Nijjar

Endometriosis the Destroyer

Endometriosis destroyer of women
Endometriosis the destroyer of the body and mind
Endometriosis the destroyer from inside out
Endometriosis the destroyer of who I am
Endometriosis the destroyer makes you a liar
Endometriosis the destroyer who judges who you are or
what you can do
Endometriosis the destroyer is my controller.
Endometriosis the destroyer of all relationships
Endometriosis overpowers my life
Endometriosis is my life.

By Donna Jardine

Messy Guest

you entered made yourself at home
you didn't knock or ask to stay
just wouldn't go away

you cooried in deep inside my core
bore down into my guts
inscribed your name upon my womb

your game to stickwith me for life
arriving never leaving &
I've been grieving ever since

the baggage which you brought
as you wrapped your fibrous arms
around each organ

held them tight
blocked out the light
I was yours all yours

I couldn't bear a child &
so we've lived our life
together just we two

but though you changed the way
things might have been
I'm used to you &

do believe you've taught me
better ways to live
to meditate to eat to pace

15

after all life's not a race
in search of who knows what
so make yourself at home

you're welcome my old friend
'cause in the end I won't be leaving you
you won't be leaving me

let's be

By Kay Ritchie

(inspired by Rumi's The Guest House)

Set me free

"Endometriosis, If we could speak
I'd ask you why you make me so weak
Always with me, never saying a word
And when I speak up about you, I struggle to be heard

You're invisible to everyone else but me
Oh, how I wish others could see
The crippling pain, the tears and fears
The excruciating struggle through the years

Endometriosis, Why won't you go away
You always come back, night and day
Please, release these chains and set me free
I just want to once again be me".

By Ine-Sophie J. Berglund

Mind of Endometriosis

Devastation amongst sadness
Betrayal amongst anger
How in the hell do I walk proudly?
When my world keeps being hit and tossed
This beast it rages amongst my body tearing me to bits
All while plastering a smile upon this face
Can't allow them to see, see the pain deep within
They don't understand just how this feels like death
Wishing silently amongst the universe to take it all away.

Devastation amongst sadness
Betrayal amongst anger
How in the hell do I live this life?
When my body screams at me over and over
This beast it rages amongst my insides murdering them
All while tears beg to be let out
Can't allow them to know, know how hurtful this is
They wouldn't understand even if I explained the pain
Wishing silently amongst the universe to be normal again.

Devastation amongst sadness
Betrayal amongst anger
How in the hell did I get here?
When trying to heal was the ultimate goal
This beast destroying everything from day one of its attack
All while pretending nothing has changed
Can't allow them inside, inside to see the damage done
They wouldn't survive the adaption forced upon me
Wishing silently amongst the universe to be pain free.

By Frosty Knoll

The Monster Who Lives Inside of Me

There is something that has taken over me,
It's crawled inside and done its worst to me,
It's truly left a curse on me.

It will pull, pinch and twist at me,
It will punch, stab and kick at me,
It will make me bleed and make me sick.

Playing little games within my mind,
Whispering that I'm lazy inside,
I question, am I crazy in my mind?

Camouflaging so well, others will question its presence
as well,
As I look so well
They have no idea of this secret hell.

It's grown, expanded, and multiplied,
Creating an epidemic inside,
Spreading far and wide.

I will never be rid of this thing,
But the world will never see,
The monster who lives inside of me.

By Beth Cooper

The Stroke of Serendipity

Spirits are intact,
Despite the devastation.
For she can weather any storm,
That's an innate fact.
An advocate with elucidation,
As her purpose takes form.

Fuelled by a dismissed reality
Standing in vulnerability
Healing through knowledge
After endometriosis almost pushed her of the ledge.

For the darkest of depths
to which she has been,
the highest of heights
and brightest of lights
await to be seen.
And perhaps that's
s e r e n d i p i t y

By Ashlee Britt Rollins

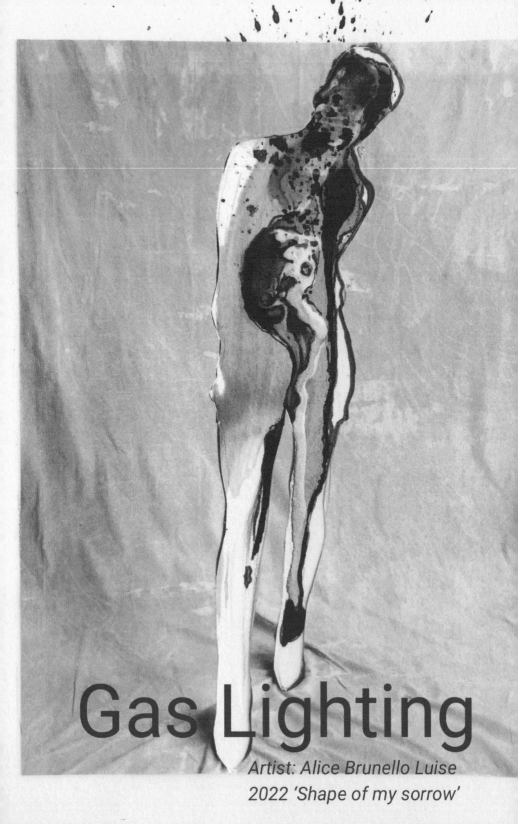

Gas Lighting

Artist: Alice Brunello Luise
2022 'Shape of my sorrow'

Dr Dr

Dr. Dr. I'm in so much pain, surely, it's not normal to feel this way.
That's just period pains, take paracetamol and be on your way.

Dr. Dr. the pain won't go away, surely, it's not normal to feel this way.
That's just period pains, use a hot water bottle and be on your way.

Dr. Dr. the pain won't go away, surely, it's not normal to feel this way.
That's just period pains, take some stronger pain killers and be on your way.

By Rachael Hird-Smith

Haunted

I am haunted,
but not by a ghost.
It's the name of a lion not so magnificent.
It's the blue eyes that linger in my dreams, turn nightmare.
It's the limp in my step,
the pain down my spine,
the droopy right eye
The images flashing,
the voice never ending,
the blood that bled.
It was my weakest moments I am haunted by.
No fault to my own,
I was sick,
diseased,
unknowingly
I was broken when I already couldn't stand.
7 years, not a day goes by I'm not haunted.
I'm reminded when I'm thriving, feeling good one day then pushing too far the next,
just to be drowned in the ghost of permanence
You may be gone but the pain is not,
the visuals are not,
the sickness is not.
You didn't' beat it out of me, you just made me worse.
You added to the negligence of no one listening to me before you knew me.

You knew of the hospital stays and the doctor visits,
you just weren't aware of the depth.
Neither was I, until now
But that's no excuse.
Overtime my weakest days showed me who was really senile.
I crawled.
I hobbled.
I bleed my way out.
I had a few hands to start to lead the way.
Knowing they saw things but just wouldn't say.
Both parents adored those hurtful hands, even if it was their own neck.
One literally, the other not as much, they helped fix my car to help see me on my way.
Knuckles red and white barely able to walk, I went back to my mother.
After some time, I found my voice, I went back to the Drs and stood my ground.
I stopped letting others walk all over me, straight down to my family.
I'm stuck not being able to pursue what I want.
Physically there isn't much flexibility.
As my back falls apart, a bigger back bone grows in its place, starting with my voice.
I am haunted, but not by a ghost.
It's the name of a lion, not so magnificent.

By Chelsea BreeAnn Hardesty

I Am Not the End

Do you hear my pleas, pain
wracking my body, endless destruction trail
behind blood lines that haunt me between my legs
I scream at the ghosts of vomit and ridicule.
Have you any mercy, pain
searing me alive, a bodice made of cysts and scars
stitched together by cells of my lost child
I held onto hope as I held this body marred.
What of my resilience, pain
never stopping, so, too, the will to fight on
another day dawns another test
I am tired, but I am not the end.

By Jessie Jing

(in response to Surita Mogan's story)

Life with Endometriosis

It's just a bad period they say, but this can't be normal no way!

When I am doubled over in pain crying on the floor, thinking I just can't take this anymore.

Doctors repeatedly gaslight you and lie, while looking you straight in the eye, telling you it's all in your head. Then why do I spend my days feeling like I am dying in bed?

When the pain feels like your insides are being twisted and ripped out, you bleed through your clothes with pain that makes you dizzy and pass out.

Finally, you find a doctor who willing to listen, and isn't brainwashed by this misogynistic healthcare system.

You go into surgery excited to finally live a life of less pain, your organs get unstuck, but you might also lose some along the way. Sadly, the joy is short lived, and your symptoms soon return, has the procedure all been in vain?

We do everything we can to manage our symptoms, cut out gluten, dairy, take 100s of supplements and so many prescriptions.

Endo so many things you have taken, causing infertility and problems with intimacy it's beyond heart breaking. We must rise-up and campaign to create more awareness to improve woman's health for our future generations.

By Gemma Starvis

The aching womb

An aching womb cries.
Relief is years away.
She is alone now.

By Sharon Teji

The Storm you Ignore

I warned you of the storm brewing in me
The untold damage disrupting my tranquillity
Gasping for air, I'm trapped in a cyclone you refuse to
see
Your ignorance was clear as day
Ignoring the warning signs to be

Standing in the eye of the storm
No one can hear me scream
Begging for a defence to defend my beaten core
Before the turbulence takes hold of me
But you ruled with assumptions, that were never to be

Your clouded judgement took hold of me
Empowering the storm encompassing me
You stole my trust
Snatching a refuge from me
Leaving me in this darkness to be

Barrowing down waiting for an end
I stumbled across a fortress of a friend
A price to pay for a calmer storm
My wounds were tended
The debris were cleared

I trusted I was saved from my fears
Which soon turned to tears
As the serpents mocked me
From the stones that misguide Hermes
Drowning Aceso within the storm

By Verity Kerr -Morrall

29

The Things They Said

"Your hips just aren't flexible enough to let baby through".
Is what they told me aged 31,
After thirty-six agonising hours,
Before they afforded me the luxury of a c-section so I could meet my beautiful baby boy.

"I'm not even referring you to gynae, my daughter died when she was 19 and you shouldn't make decisions like that about the future".
Is what the Nurse Practitioner told me aged 32,
After telling her I knew I would never have another child and I wanted those parts of me gone.
My son made me complete, and childbirth had been my trauma.

"Let's try you with the coil if you don't like the pill".
Said the Sexual Health Nurse when I was 32.
Little did I know how painful that would be until I was writhing around,
Or vomiting most weeks.

"I've referred you to the team who help with painful sex".
Said the Doctor when I went to see him aged 33.
I'd told him that any sex for me meant excruciating pain on my right,
From my bowel to my ovaries.

"I'm just going to have a feel up here, you don't mind my male colleague watching do you. He's in training"
Said the woman at the clinic when I was 34.
Just before she prescribed me 5 plastic phalluses of varying sizes,
To help "open me up".

"I know the migraines are linked to my cycle".
I said maybe 50 times to various Doctors.
When I wasn't losing whole days of my life having them,
Unable to go to work or play with my son.

"I'm so bloated and its agony to go to the loo. I have to pant while I'm going!"
I told the Doctor aged 35.
Just before he referred me to the bowel clinic,
For an internal camera.

"There's nothing wrong inside your bowel".
Said the consultant smugly.
Just as he thought, no doubt,
I was just being silly.

"I think you're probably just having an early menopause".
Said the Nurse Practitioner with a chuckle in her voice,
On my twentieth call to the GP surgery aged 36
"I'm not" I cried softly to myself.

"You can see our locum Doctor today".
Said the receptionist on my next call, aged 37.
"Yes please" I said.
"I think you need a referral to Gynae" he said.

"I can't bear it" I screamed.
As I lay on the floor, a massage ball under my right-hand side.
Trying to ease the pressure,
Waiting for my appointment.

"I think I need an ambulance" I cried down the phone to my Mum.
I can't get up off the floor.
I can't stay awake.
The pain is too much!

"The Camera shows nothing on the inside".
Said the consultant . . . but you can't see Endometriosis unless you have a laparoscopy.
"I'll book you in" he said to me, aged 38.

"Everything's stuck together, you're covered in it".
Said my consultant, as I came around from the operation in a daze.
"I told you, I told everyone" I cried.
But no-one could hear me.

"This is the top Endometriosis consultant in the County".

He said, just a few weeks before I met my hero.
He knows everything about Endometriosis.
"Here's the next battle", I thought.

"You have Stage 4 Endometriosis".
Said the Gynae Surgeon to me aged 40.
It's the worst it can be,
"Your bladder, your bowel, your uterus, they're all stuck"

"No one has listened to me for all these years".
I sobbed, a grown woman.
"Please take it all away. My womb, my ovaries, everything"
"I can do that for you," said my hero.

"It was a success.
"We managed to scrape it off your bowel without damaging it".
"You don't need a colostomy bag".
"Your bowel will revert to its normal shape".
"Your ovaries have been removed".
"Your womb has been removed".
"Your bladder is unstuck".

You're free.
And I finally was, aged 41

By Claire Chapman

Time passes

Time passes
The pain does not.
Hours spent advocating for something you're told will be taken care of.
Health.
Your health
When it's in jeopardy only then do you discover the broken system, you're a part of.
Waitlists: sometimes years long, you try to be patient...
but you want to scream
"Why won't anyone listen to me?"
This is not normal.
The list of symptoms are never ending, you start to doubt your own reality.
"Maybe it's unrelated."
Testing
Testing
Poking
Prodding
Inconclusive.
"Results look normal."
Although you know something is wrong. Something deeper.

Finally, a specialist who listens. Except he's over 9000 km, 3 flights, 2 continents away.
You travel to meet him.
For relief
For your life back
For a chance at "normalcy"

Your surgery is complex. 4.5 hours. Advanced stage 4
endometriosis.
Your surgery is a success.
8 months have passed.
Your recovery: a long, tumultuous road.
Your journey: almost incomprehensible now, feels like a
windswept dream.

Moments, memories, sensations of the past creep
forward.

How can this be? A piece of the "old you" is back.
Integrating your lived trauma into your "new normal".
Fear.
Always present.
"What if the disease grows back?"
"What if my relief is only temporary?"
"Why do I still feel pain?"
Time passes
The pain does not.

By Sydney Doberstein Larock

Valentine's Day

I used to watch her crawl
Hear her vomit after eating
Watch her pass out in the kitchen
Hear her cry in agony
And I always worried
Because how would I ever help
If I didn't know what it was
And she didn't either.

My mum is the best mum
While she raised us
Multiple organs were covered
Strangling her
And she would still laugh and love us

When we said goodbye
I thought I'd see her later that day
But the call didn't come
For hours
I watched the clock, the phone, the window
It wasn't routine after all
It was an emergency
Six hours
Stage IV

And we were never knew
But she came home on Valentine's Day
And it was the best one yet
Because now we knew
It was all real

By Lorna Merrow

Flare up
Artist: Iness Rychlik

Barbed Wire Body

Coils of steel embedded in pelvis
scraping organs at every turn,
a shriek, static, a portrait of pain,
mask shattered in broken glass shards.

As the barbed wire chokes, let me breathe,
I will endure as I always do,
do not make me hide this quaking pain,
showing my discomfort shreds malignant apathy.

By Tori Pearmain

Counting Tiles

Counting bathroom tiles while the pain won't quit,
Each month, I mark them, an unchanging number.
I stay put in here, I won't get up.
Blood is easier to clean,
From tiles than bedsheets.

Dizziness spins, tiles dance,
Can't stand tall,
I don't even bother to try.
I won't budge,
This bathroom is my own little retreat,
Alone with my pain, no one else around.

Once a moon, in here, I spend my days alone.
Loneliness and isolation is what I know,
The tiles see it all, a monthly fight.
Solitude and pain are my companions,
They know me well.

Sometimes I leave but I'll always come back,
Behind this bathroom door,
A save haven,
A prison,
A sanctuary,
To count the tiles.

By Liz Van Ingen

Escape

Another place
Another world
An escape I crave

Yet I'm cradled by the
cold, pearl, porcelain

Caressed by the
unsympathetic tile floor

An odd sense of comfort here
An all in one
in home
escape

Not the one I crave

By Chelsea BreeAnn Hardesty

It's just period pain

Every month, the same sequence
Never ending fear of the pain to come
Debilitating, life altering pain
Over the counter medications won't touch it

Making excuse after excuse
Every month, the same routine
Trying to hold your life together

Reaching for anything that might help the pain
Indescribable guilt for letting people down
Only to be told that this is normal
Sacrificing relationships, jobs, and friendships

Insisting that there is something wrong
Suffering cause 'every woman goes through it'
This is not just period pain, this is our lives, our reality
with endometriosis

By Leona McKenzie

Hand to endo belly

heavy as a sack of sugar sticky tricky
a maze of convoluted chocolate cysts & ovaries that kiss

a labyrinth where bull-like creatures
rampage rage wage war

heavy hooves & no respect
they charge at flaming fibroids

gnaw at thick adhesions
strangling my baby

inside tangled tubes
tears turn red &

tumble like the waterfalls
of all the blood I've lost

these beasts are furious &
my womb doesn't work

my breasts become suck-dry &
I accept I'll never have this child

I'll never have another
I'll never be a mother

By Kay Ritchie

I See Red

I see red.

The relief, the scream into the pillow.
The wave is gone.
A break, gushing down it comes
Like a dam that's exploded and broken
into tiny pieces.

I see red.

Each piece is different, it's own alien-like
shape- rounder, clumpier, smaller and larger.
But they're all the same- a haunting image
that will not go away. When will it end?
When will it be different?

I see red.

It's invaded. It's taken control.
Growing inside and spreading out - poison!
The clumps of hair on the floor,
the TV still on from the night before,
the pills on the table which have not worked,
and the sorry sight of stained clothes
that remain hung in the closet to air.
Clothes I'll never wear again -
Scrub, scrub, scrub - it won't go away!
Haunted by the present and the past.

I see red.

By Christine

Rage

Give me a stage.
I will rage.
Allow me to raise my pitch.
Burn b...

By Hana Buchalíková Bujňáková

Suffering

Suffering
Best kept secret
Ashamed
In pain
Alone
Misunderstood issues
Embarrassed
Uncomfortable with you

By Antje Bothin

Where have you been?

I have been in bed.
Under my heating pad.
I have been crying.
In the emergency room.
Waiting in waiting rooms.
Riding in the back of my mom's car trying not to throw
up.
I have been alone.
I have been exhausted, but not sleeping.
I have been on the floor of my shower
With hot water pouring overtop of me.
I have been over my toilet.
Throwing up.
Tears streaming down my face.
Where have I been?
Well, you see I've been in pain.

By Sheridan T

Surgery

Artist: Clare Gregory
X Marks the Spot

Diagnosis E

The Pain-
Trickles down my skin,
Deep within.
These fibroids-
Mesh from head to toe.
My body cannot create,
Cannot withhold my hate.
My balance and my self-belief.
Keep me cold and without desire.
This situation is withholding my fight.
My words, not my actions
Cannot withstand motivation.
Or blame,
Keeps me tame.
My distant heart bleeds tears.
You take away my happiness.
Like a pin, I swallow and withhold my faith.
I scream 'I shout'
Please let me out!
Another op, will it be successful?
The myth, the madness.
Just talk about your fears,
Let's shout-the road must go somewhere.
Let out your woes,
In every breath.
It feels heavy, my side hurts.
You've taken away my fertility.
What it means to be me.

Just let me be-
Let it ease-
Let me succeed!
Not to live to please,
What did I do to endure?
When I cannot anymore.
Did I do something awful?
In a past life? That aside-
Let me make an apology.
Let things change,
So, I can learn to live another day.

By Nisha Pearson

Imagine

Imagine for a minute your diagnosed with endometriosis!

Imagine for a minute the excruciating cramps that searing through your body.

Imagine for a minute the sleepless painful nights.

Imagine for a minute the sensation of electric shock bursting throughout your pelvis.

Imagine for a minute being sent home during a flare-up by A&E with no treatment, symptom, or pain relief.

Imagine for a minute being bounced around the NHS from department to department with no treatment plan.

Imagine for a minute that your symptoms are gas lighted by every single medical professional you see.

Imagine for a minute that surgery will be a regular occurrence for symptom management.

Imagine for a minute being unable to complete a working week.

Imagine for a minute that there is no cure.

Imagine this is your life!

By Charley Cutter

In the quiet realm of my existence

In the quiet realm of my existence, pain became an unwelcome companion, a relentless shadow that refused to release its grip. Endometriosis, the silent creator of my suffering, wove its intricate web within me, an incurable disease that carved pathways of torment through the very core of my being.

Countless surgeries, each one a battlefield where skilled hands fought against an adversary unseen. The operating table became a temporary respite, a brief intermission in a symphony of agony. As the scars multiplied, so did the echoes of resilience, etching a narrative of battles waged and fortitude found in the midst of the surgeon's sterile theatre.

The sterile scent of hospitals and the rhythmic beeping of machines became the backdrop to a life defined by the unpredictable dance of pain.

Each surgery held the promise of relief, a hope that proved elusive, slipping through my grasp like grains of sand.

et, in the quiet aftermath of surgical storms, there emerged a phoenix of strength from the ashes of despair. The scars on my body became a testimony to survival, a roadmap of endurance etched in the language of surgical stitches. As I navigated the maze of medical uncertainty, the whispers of my spirit echoed louder than the ache within.

Endometriosis, an uninvited guest in the ballroom of my life, could not extinguish the dance of my indomitable spirit. With every surgery, I embraced the uncertainty, stitching resilience into the very fabric of my existence. In the shadow of incurable affliction, I found the strength to endure, to persist, and to craft a narrative of bravery in the face of relentless pain.

By Cassandra Nordal

Invisible to See

They say it's invisible to see.
Unless you're a magician to be.

I have a mission for you to see.
The vision of endometriosis to be.

The clinician brought me to tears.
Due to the omission of my fears.

Demolished by their unawares.
Ooh, how I wished they would care.

Why can't they repair …
Invisible belittled me.

By Verity Kerr -Morrall

It Finds a Way

A cocktail as a reminder
Another one needed
The foulness
As it sets in for release
Preparation for excavation
Of a returning disease
No matter
It finds a way

Reappearing like magic
Taking root
Devouring, like a picnic
The same white cold room
Repeated direction
Sharp pinch
Preparing way to unearth
A recurrent condition
It finds a way

Through the hallways
Into the elevator
Feeling, fuzzy, colder
Machines beep
Familiar voices
Oxygen mask holders
Nothing, then awake
From the reprise
Of an unending affliction
As it always
Finds a way

By Chelsea BreeAnn Hardesty

Laparoscopy, 1992

(i.m. – Frida Kahlo, 1907 – 1945)

now I have a name for it
after all the years
misdiagnosed
labelled
offered pills
I have a name
after years of
sleeplessness
chronic pain
fatigue
neglect &
flare ups
I have a name
it has a name
and I am not alone
I am woman &
like Frida Kahlo I will live
around it with it through it
let it shapeshift into
images & colours
let it flow let it go
let it grow into words
transported to the page
which holds it
makes it real
let's me feel

that I'm not mad
as doctors often said
and oh the pain
the pain of being woman
being so misunderstood
the pain that teaches
womanhood
gratitude
this pain
which has a name
is mine
I'll grow to love it

By Kay Ritchie

Scars

The scars forced upon me.
A timeline you see.
Where excision had to be.

An artist at work.
Sculpting the lesions away.
Leaving their mark in the way.

My canvas signed with a stich.
A scar created for me.
A memory of A dream to be.

By Verity Kerr -Morrall

(Inspired by Clare Gregory's 'endometriosis belly buttons'.)

Tears

T they said you must be mistaken; you cannot
be in that much pain!

E eventually, as things get worse, years go by,
they decide to take a look.

A all over, they find endo, quick look becomes
six hours. Complicated is what they say.

R recovery, where to begin, unknown. Now it is
gone, what is left?

S support – where is it? After care? Silence. Is it
really gone?

By Georgina Moon

Womber 5/6/1977 – 16/7/2018

Wombs are very important,
I used to have one as well.

We started off just fine,
Then she drove me to hell.

Gifting me two beautiful children,
She did just swell.

She then got pissed,
So I got rid.

I named her 'Womber'

After all the blood and tears,
I will not miss her.

I looked forward to happier years,
But that wasn't meant for me.

As endo had it in for me!

By Aine Drummond

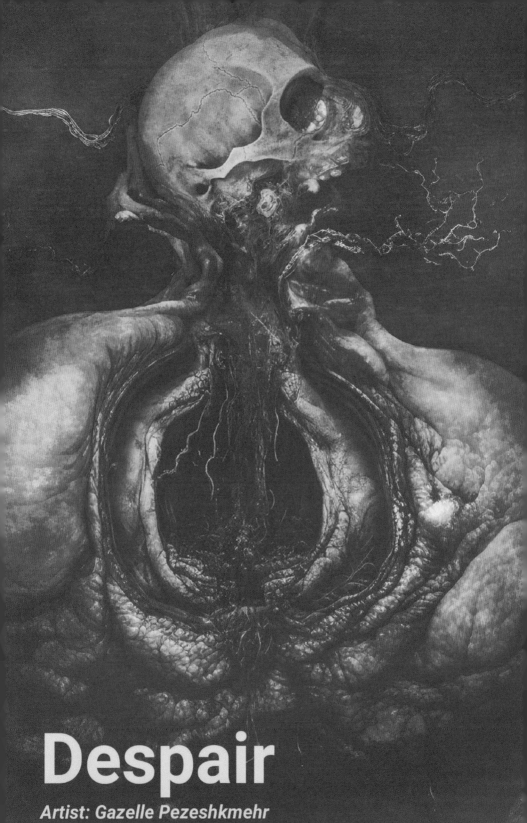

Despair

Artist: Gazelle Pezeshkmehr

A Lifetime of Medical Debt by the Age of 25

I cried on my way to infusions / had to stop half way to the building, leaning heavy on my rollator / wept again in the bathroom / pulled my phone from my pocket / is it my essential tremor or the fact my eyes are swimming making my screen impossible to read? / I voice memo incoherencies / the pain is claws cracking my hips / electric poles piercing my bladder / I am stepping on nails and my back hasn't stopped spasming / I think it's time to go back under the knife / can we even afford a fifth opinion? / a third surgery? / how are we planning on paying off the last one? / I need to do something other than fucking breathing so I am researching people who perform laparoscopies from my seat at the infusion clinic / I finally reeled in my emotions with action / you message me / we will do whatever we have to in order to get the pain down! / I'm hoping you catch a break soon / please drive safe / I waste my hydration / sobbing over a text / to love and be loved by you / is one of the few reasons I can keep going

By Maggie Bowyer

Am I Worthy

If I told you my story would you listen?
Would there be compassion or care?
Am I worthy?

Conquering season after season
Passionately present
In moments promised
Yet fading

Uncompassionate noise
Attempting to drown,
At the end of the rope
There was hope

Reflection, perspective, confidence
Silencing the noise, then trust
Through healing eyes
Through protective guidance

God allowed my eyes to see
How he saw me
Am I worthy?

God fuelled me
Otherwise I'd be destroyed
A purpose to speak on

You are not alone
Life has purpose
You're equipped for every season
You are worthy

By Chelsea BreeAnn Hardesty

(Inspired by a short story submitted to project 514 415)

As You Depart for The Stars

As you depart for the stars
carry me with you
Traverse the universe
Findthe brightest heavenly body
and lie to rest—
—therewe will meet one day
whence the future becomes past.

For though a cloudy night veils
the celestial from the earthly
Your heavenly body remains
Away from the terrestrial
tethered eternally—
—heart, soul, and mind
ablaze and alive.

Hope is like a star in the sky
may not be seen but always there
For only time will tell
And as you depart
soon to become a star—
—Hope, my dear baby
Farewell.

By Jessie Jing

Broken Soul

Wishing for death beneath my breath
Dark as the night
Not a constructive thought in sight

Life's plain purpose is sterile
Lonely, rural, bordering on feral

No more naivety
Banished productivity
For I have no desire for longevity

Take me home
To where I actually belong
Wishing for death
Beneath my breath

Take me home
Let's not sugar coat or honey comb
To the peaceful divine darkness
soothing my spiritual catharsis

Presented as the family matriarch
Self representation - depicted no more than a decaying
carcass
A former shell of ones self

To hell with mental health
Not even a skelp
Could self assure myself

For I am wishing death beneath my breath
Swiftly hurled into the next world
Longing for surpass
In my after worldly forecast

By Stacey Smith

Helpless

I feel helpless inside.
As she tries to hide
The agonising pain
She battles night and day.

I can do the chores.
And try to offer support.
Hold her hand in her fight.
Hug her extra tight.

But I can't take endometriosis away.
I can't get rid of the pain.
That I watch her face day by day
I now know what those with Endo face.

By Aimee Gill

(Inspired by a short story submitted to project 514 415)

Pain, a work
in progress

It's the beating of a drum against my back,
my thighs trickling with sweat
as I am battered by nerves
my throat constricted
around a void

No, it's-
Stinging nettles and hawthorn
grazing my skin raw and raging
at every touch until
I'm clammed in heat
and have to rest

No, it's-
Choking as lightning cracks my bones
and thunder roils in my belly
as I step outside and run
last appointment's outcome
my body rejects it

No, it's-
Losing feeling, limb by limb
struggling to think, to listen
brain turning, shuddering shut
the nut and bolt stuck
jarring my teeth

No, it's-
Sticking my face in metal pins
wearing a mask tight compressed
struggling for breath
my body hemmed in
frame of wire mesh

No, it's-
Knocking on the door with the metal plaque
arms cramping, legs barely standing
just hoping for better, for more, for less
that I'll express my pain under duress
stand my ground whilst my heart pounds
explain myself again and again
the pain is ten out of ten
do you believe me
will you treat me
I wait for you to say
"Come in"

By Tori Pearmain

slow and steady

slow and steady
wins the race
right?
i'm not sure who i'm against
all i see is me
crawling to the finish line
full of chronic pain

but,

the finish line
just keeps just getting further away
maybe it will all become clear
one day

By Saskia Ayre

The Robber

I am exhausted, I long for sleep, for a release out of this hellish prison I call my body, yet I know there will be no escape. I leave the safety of my bed and head downstairs. Morphine, pills, heaty Harry, this routine is as normal to me as breathing.

I can't give in; I WON'T give in! Endometriosis has robbed so much from me, so many moments with my children, my soulmate stolen, reducing me to a mere watcher, a stalker on my family's lives.

Operation after operation, robbing my body of the home I grew my babies, of what makes me a woman, certainly by societies standards. But it won't win, I'll keep fighting.

By Kirsty Clarke

What if

but
what if
what if there are no answers
what if
what if this is my life now

uncomfortable
in pain
i will do anything
to just make it all go away

By Saskia Ayre

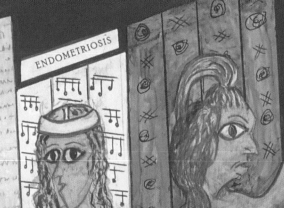

ENDOMETRIOSIS

Support

Artist: Terrence Conway

Endo Advocate

Endo :: Endo :: Endo :: Endo

:: Endo :: Endo :: Endo :: Endo :: Endo

:: Endo :: Endo :: Endo :: Endo

Endo from a mothers eyes

Watching your child living in so much pain,
Not able to fix it, oh what a shame!
Breathing through cramps like she's in labour,
Me feeling like such a bloody failure.

Doctors don't listen,
"Endo is rare in children".
"Take paracetamol and go to school",
Thanks for that, so very unhelpful.

Finally finding someone who'll listen,
Watching her eyes start to glisten.
First surgery undergone at just fourteen,
Endo confirmed for my beautiful teen.

"We have a support group, but you're too young",
This journey feels like it's just begun.
Six years and one more surgery later,
Her body has become such a traitor.

She has done so much to help other people,
Whilst preparing again for her own next sequel.
Friendships lost and new ones made,
From within a community, she wants to aid.

Such a strong woman who stands apart,
My Child
My Daughter
The beat of my heart.

By Emma Gill

Life

How do you feel, when you start the day?
An ache, some soreness, does it soon go away?

Do you open an eye, and hope for the best?
Or do you want to cry, because you just need to rest?

I see you asleep, and smile to myself.
The only part of the day, you feel in good health.

But then you wake, and the pain takes hold.
Etched on your face, making you feel old.

You need your pills, they give light relief.
You'd beg for some more but you'd feel like a thief.

Composing yourself, you start your day.
Deep down hoping the pain will be taken away.

But that's only a dream, can never come true.
So getting on with your life is all you can do.

I want to feel it, wish I could take it away.
Free you from hell, even just for one day.

I see you in tears, exhausted from living.
Pain crushing you down, it's always winning.

The night finally enters, soon to be sleeping.
I hold you close for that's when I do my weeping.

Holding you close protecting from the pain
But tomorrow will come and you'll do it all again.

By Stewart Craigon

Lost and Not Found

And she cried with a pain
that cut deeper and deeper
year after year
until she was no more.
Lost and not found
my Endometriosis warrior.
Suffering a profound,
endless without sound thing,
a no light to be found thing,
may the darkness not spread-out thing
We pray for no more cruelties of the
Medically unsound things.
Let's cause not more doubting,
And find this out, please.

By Cameron Hardesty

Speak Up

I woke up one day and everything changed
Life before that day now seems so strange
The pain gets so intense that I double in two
What is this pain? I wish I knew

People say "speak up speak up don't cry alone"
But oh how I wish this pain would go
"Speak up speak up now don't be scared"
But I just wish I could be repaired

I'm sad all the time almost every day
Chronic pain every day how can I be this way?
I miss so much school, this makes me lose friends
And catching up on work never seems to end

Months are now years and tears are now fears
But I still don't know why my pain is so severe
So much pain but I'm so young
I just miss the days when I got things done

I'll never be cured, I know I'll have good days and bad
But being ill all the time makes me so mad
So I'm gonna speak up speak up I won't cry alone
I'll speak up speak up and I won't be scared

By Aimee Gill

Spoon Theory

Lie stiff and stretched out like an effigy
In bed, caved in, completely given up,
Lie flat out, long lost like a refugee
Need saving from myself, lost any backup

Wish I backed up, said stop a while ago
When I had the chance, seen where it would lead
Now abandoned to pain that's to the bone
In spoon debt, can't do what's a basic need

Forgo washing up for urgent repair,
Charge battery not just drained but broken
To maybe cook meal, no energy spared
For friends waiting with plans left unspoken

They enjoy spoon surplus, I only dream
Curled into myself with my body's scream

By Joy Getliffe

The body's waltz

A cool touch settles on heated skin
White streaks interweave red patches
Reminiscent of flames burning within
A phœnix rises from its ashes.

Scars are residences of memories
Bygone states materialised onto surface
Within and through this vessel of corporeality
Presence-absence interlaces.

Heed the call of the pulse
A symphony existing beneath the skin
Of which we shall call The Body's Waltz
I dance to and live for over and over again.

These fingers trace the body's flux and flow
Between the pain and sheer will we find hope.

By Jessie Jing

The Enchanted Circle

Oh, the enchanted circle of those who stand by us in our trials.

The ones who lift us up from the abyss of surgeries, offer us warmth with their heat packs, soothe our souls by washing our faces, and stay with us throughout the night.

To our partners, who embrace us with boundless love, holding us as we weep,
whispering words of hope when pain overwhelms us, seeing the perfectness within us even in our darkest moments.

To the women who bear the weight of their suffering in silence, shrouded in shame and fear of failure.

To the pain that threatens to engulf us, suffocating us and consuming our spirits. And yet, within our tiny bodies, we find the courage to fight, to persevere, to flourish.
Our bodies are our allies, whispering to us when something is amiss, cheering us on when we achieve a victory.

To the doctors who turned us away with no answers, and to those who listened and aided in our recovery, we are grateful.

To the women who fight daily for their right to live in peace, to those who wake up every day in pain yet go to work anyway, and to those who love the world even when it feels
unbearable.

To those who endure the heartache, heartbreak, and suffering of others, to the moments of light that shine through the darkness, and to the life force of femininity that fuels us all.

By Deneika Klynnyk

The Moon and a Body out of Orbit

The Goddess Selene drives the moon through the sky in
Greece.
When I was there, I spoke to a couple
(she was Italian, he was German)
Who said that for her the moon is feminine, for him
masculine.
I reflected on this months later when lying in an attic
in Wales, where the moon is called lleuad.
Here most of us are moon-faced, here where the sun
pales much more than in southern Europe, most
certainly
compared to the Northeast of Africa, to Egypt
where I grew as a teenage girl discovering menstruation
and developing endometriosis, under the wholesome
gaze
of alqamar. Its spermy light dazzled upon
infinitesimal grains; making a mother out of the desert,
making a future question of my being a mother

By Helen Grant

Would you stay?

Would you stay by my side if you knew?
Knew that I had been cursed by a disease that cannot be
lifted.

Would you plan a future with me if our plans may just be
a fantasy?
Fantasying about a family that may never be.

Would you be angry if I cancelled and headed to bed?
Bedded by pain, nausea, and fatigue.

Would you wipe my tears and hold me tight?
Tight enough to make my fears disappear.

Would you be by myside when I awake from surgery?
Surgery that may not be the last.

Would you grow to hate me for the disruption of
endometriosis?
Endometriosis that took hold of me.

By Verity Kerr -Morrall

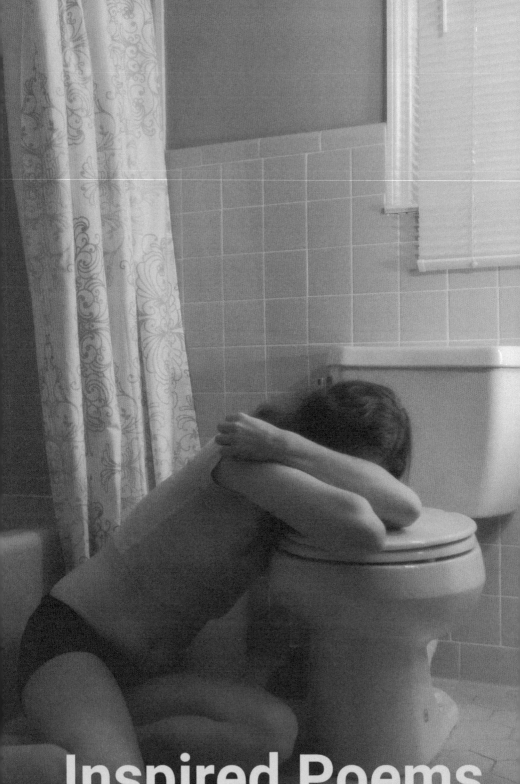

Inspired Poems
Artist: Charlotte Montgomery

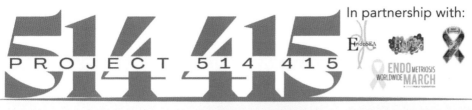

BURN BITCH

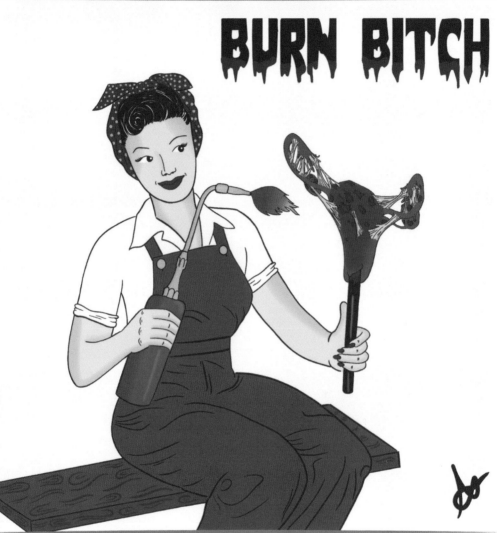

Endometriosis has been found on every single organ in the body, not just the reproductive system

www.project 514 415.com
Sharing the Lived Experiences of Endometriosis

Burn, burn

On a cold bed, in a sterilised room,
a bonfire was lit in my body,
tissue torched by a hand
wielding diathermic tools.

I want it to burn,
that flesh, deliverer of pain,
but I do not want to be burned,
like a wilted rose under a looking glass.

I imagine my hand scorching flesh
then throwing the memory of pain
riddled organs in a can
and giving them a trial by fire.

By Tori Pearmain

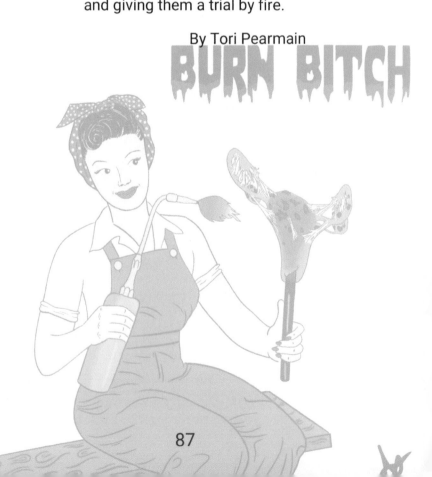

BURN BITCH

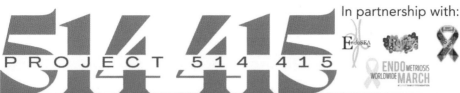

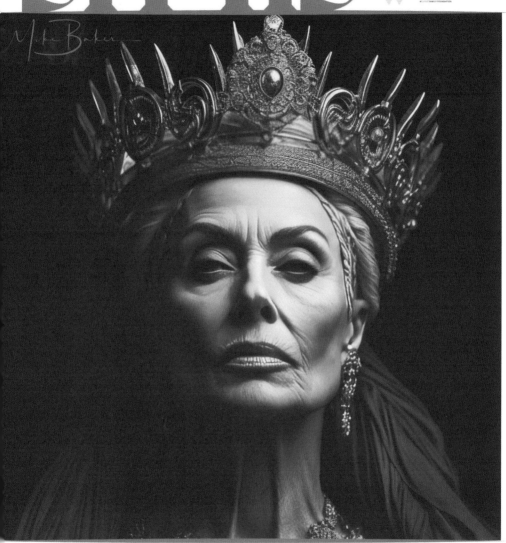

Endometriosis continues to impact people
after menopause and / or a hysterectomy

The Eyes

A window to the soul,
they tell a tale.
The years like mountains,
overcoming the deadliest peaks.
Her words,
strict, poised, structured, precise.
A life guided on instilled principles,
normal dispositional.

Generational Damage
Begetting Confusion

What could she do?
Propagated centennial ideals,
withheld paths to answers.
For her. For them. For they. For all.
Past. Present. Future.
Our ancestors wondering,
why and how many more?

What can we do?
Rise up. Speak up. Team up.
Find the strength in your journey, like they.

We all bare the marks of battles unseen,
draw from the generational wisdom.
The matched endurance,
through the turbulence.
It shall bring the crown of resilience,
to all

The cosmos may be seen,
through the eyes.
A revolution may begin,
through the voice.

By Chelsea BreeAnn Hardesty

514 415

In partnership with:

EndoSEA
ENDOMETRIOSIS WORLDWIDE MARCH

PROJECT 514 415

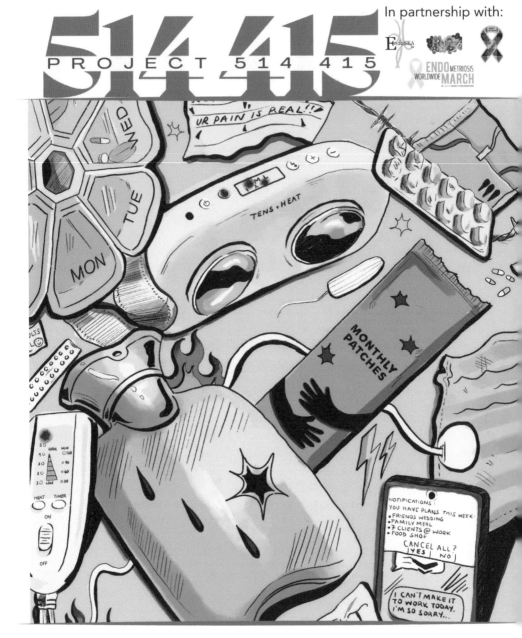

Endometriosis has no cure, only symptom management strategies which aim to reduce the symptoms caused by endometriosis.

www.project 514 415.com

Sharing the Lived Experiences of Endometriosis

Taking Over

I immediately remove the heat from my skin when I
begin to splotch into red, like a strawberry cow.

I immediately crave it again. The only thing that feels
deep enough to touch the pain.

Red, hot, searing stimulation. A distraction from the
rooted monster beneath the surface, taking over.

The stimulating vibration of the tens unit takes place, as
I await the rush of partial relief from the pills consumed.

Hoping to make scheduled plans. Scrambling to pack
the must haves. As I predict the monster beneath the
surface, taking over.

By Chelsea BreeAnn Hardesty

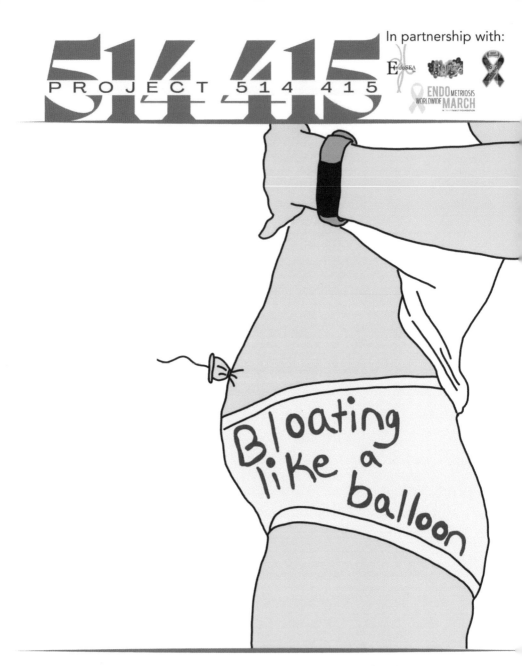

Medical imagery such as MRIs and ultrasounds can miss endometriosis lesions often resulting in being told that there is nothing wrong.

www.project 514 415.com
Sharing the Lived Experiences of Endometriosis

Nothing Wrong?

I am told there is nothing wrong.
MRIs, ultrasounds...
Nothing wrong.

Yet my belly speaks.

By Hana Buchalíková Bujňáková

Bloating like a balloon

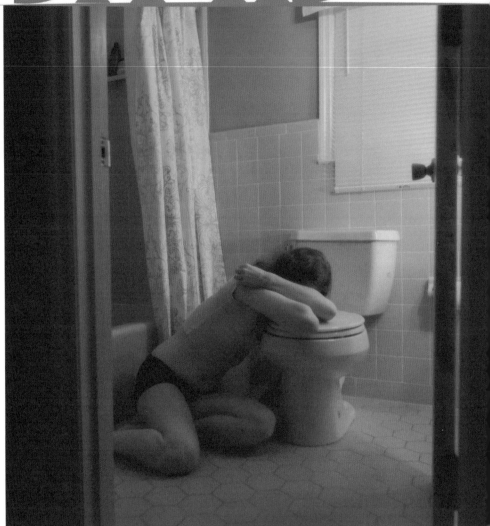

PROJECT 514 415

It can take on average 8 years to be diagnosed with endometriosis, many suffer in silence for decades until they are diagnosed.

www.project 514 415.com
Sharing the Lived Experiences of Endometriosis

Weary Head

Every moment of the day I am forced to drag myself
from bed.
The cold ceramic of the toilet basin has become a place
to rest my weary head.
Huddled, crouched on the floor, goosebumps, tiles touch
bare skin.
All whilst pain ruptures inside of me, a sensation rising
from within.

A sharp sensation, organs fusing, burning.
A sensation as though my colon is being squeezed,
something twisting and turning.
A heavy sensation pulling down on my abdomen,
causing pressure, force.
A sensation that's relentless it shows no signs of
remorse.

A deep sensation, charging, right through to my core.
A sensation as though my energy is seeping, pooling, out
onto the bathroom floor.
The time has come to pick myself up, dragging myself
back to bed.
I know that once again the toilet basin will become a
place to rest my weary head.

By Clare Gregory

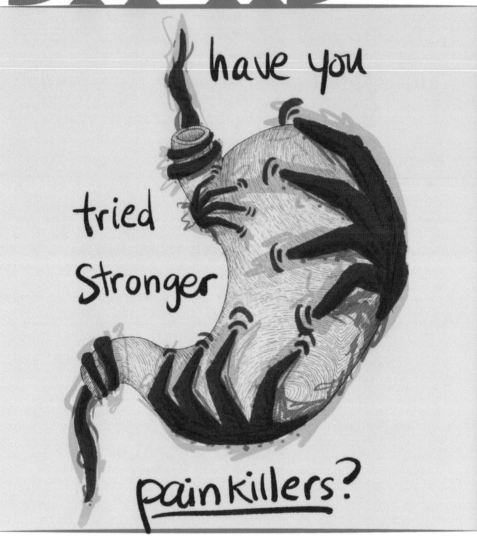

PROJECT 514 415

In partnership with:

have you tried Stronger painkillers?

The NHS listed endometriosis among the 20 most painful medical conditions, along with cancer, appendicitis and heart attack.

www.project 514 415.com
Sharing the Lived Experiences of Endometriosis

Haunting

Ghosts grip my organs,
their ghoulish laughter
ripples my torso.
I shake, made possessed.

My flesh feels monstrous,
dark shadows haunt me,
my feelings die a death.
Choked, claustrophobic, numb.

By Tori Pearmain

514 415

In partnership with:

PROJECT 514 415

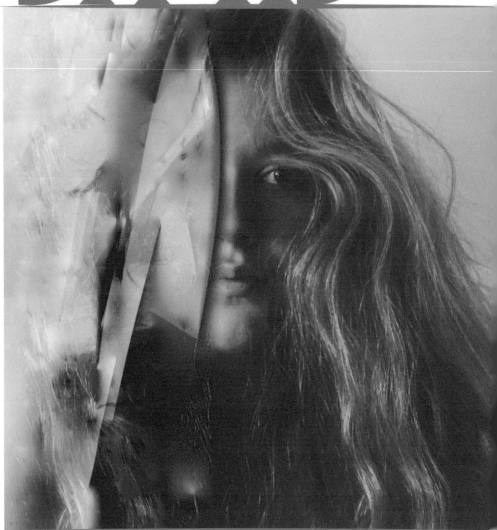

Many people with endometriosis suffer in silence with uncontrolled pain and chronic fatigue.

www.project 514 415.com

Sharing the Lived Experiences of Endometriosis

See me

Look into my eyes.
What do you see?

I may seem OK.

Being brave every day.
Going unnoticed.

Look at me.

Notice my eyes and feel how my soul pleads.
Notice how I scream.

When will this agony end?
When will someone understand?

Every day, I fight through the pain.
Every day, I squeeze out some energy to keep going.

Did you know this?

Just look into my eyes.

Look...
...and you will see.

By Hana Buchalíková Bujňáková

514 415

PROJECT 514 415

In partnership with:

EndoSEA

ENDO METRIOSIS
WORLDWIDE MARCH

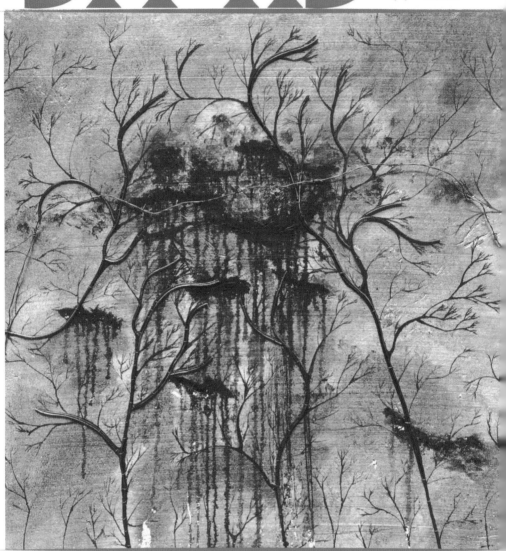

Endometriosis lesion have their own nerve fibres,
blood vessels and immune cells.

Rootbound

My womb makes roots where it shouldn't.
Red tissue entwines my ovaries encasing them,
making them rootbound, suffocated.

Strands of tissue break free, slipping out
to reach a space to breathe: my bladder,
my intestines, unknown spaces in my abdomen.

When you walk through a forest of trees,
the roots sleep underneath, the black chasm
of the soil under your feet, you know they are there
no question.

Must we rely on an imaging device
that cannot find roots
to decide whether a patient gets care?

Why are the words from the body
that can feel these roots
judged in a way that's unfair?

By Tori Pearmain

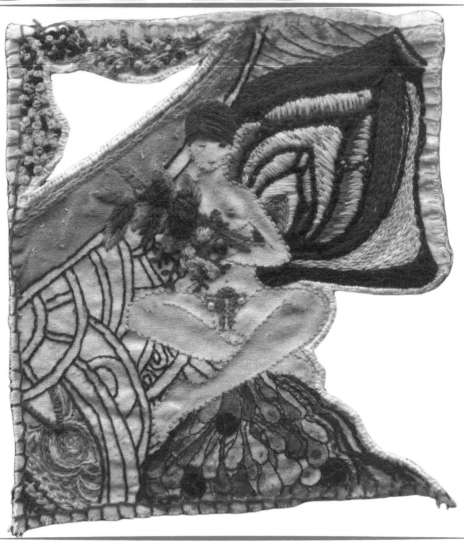

Endometriosis lesions produce
their own estrogen.

www.project 514 415.com
Sharing the Lived Experiences of Endometriosis

Amongst The Clotted Rose

Inside this walled garden I am feminine and serene,
See here the bouquet of brights within my hands,
The pearls of my womanhood, how preciously they shine.
I sit cross-legged, opening up my story to you
But across the lands beyond the uterine
My dreams and nightmares mercilessly fuse.
Here the clotted rose grows like a weed,
The pain stitched into my body in fence-like scars.
At the back of my mind
A strip of sky is lightly tinged with blue,
The chance of pregnancy passing through?
It is dotted with torn threads
From a guilt-ridden galaxy of unborn stars
But below this are virginal cells of white
And up above, just to the right,
A curious leaf grows,
A variegated one
Of purple grief and yellow hope
Showing that we are
Despite our wounds
Still women of the kaleidoscope,
Still living in colour
Even amongst the clotted rose.

By Sarah Mills

514 415

PROJECT 514 415

In partnership with:

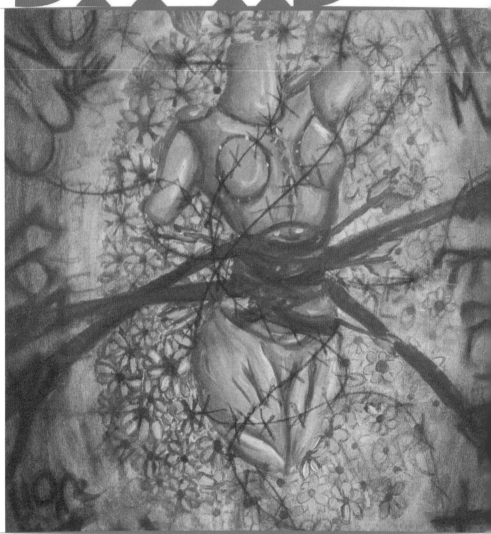

Endometriosis can cause debilitating
symptoms and secondary health concerns
when not managed.

www.project 514 415.com
Sharing the Lived Experiences of Endometriosis

Sun/Blood

Crisp buttercups and fresh daffodils
frame the brilliance of the day.
I lay, sundress splayed,
the image of feminine innocence.

Inside I am robotic, cranking
the turn of my limbs as dictated
by ribbons curled around my organs.
Bloodied tissue turns to pain turns to burnt metal.

In an upside-down world
bright sunflowers blossom inside my body,
around me the ground heaves tumultuously,
roots constrained beneath black-blooded flesh.

By Tori Pearmain

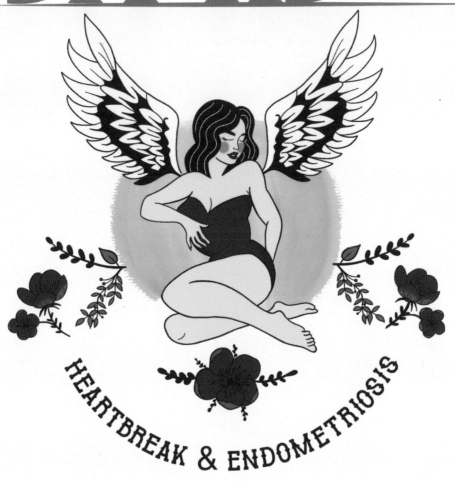

514 415

PROJECT 514 415

In partnership with:

EndoSEA

ENDOMETRIOSIS WORLDWIDE MARCH

HEARTBREAK & ENDOMETRIOSIS

@endoandme2023

Endometriosis is a inflammatory
condition where endometrium-like tissue
is found throughout the body.

www.project 514 415.com
Sharing the Lived Experiences of Endometriosis

Heartbreak

My body inflamed.
Abnormal cells may be found anywhere.

My body aches.
My heart breaks.

I am an angel who needs to stop and rest...

By Hana Buchalíková Bujňáková

514 415

In partnership with:

EndoSEA

ENDOMETRIOSIS
WORLDWIDE MARCH

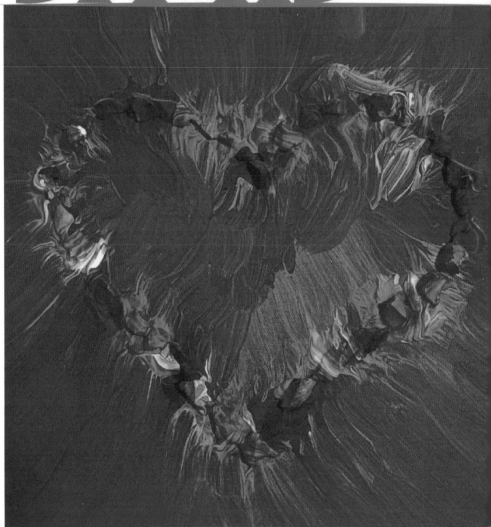

Endometriosis does not discriminate,
impacting all cultures, disabilities and
members of the LGBTQ+ community.

www.project 514 415.com
Sharing the Lived Experiences of Endometriosis

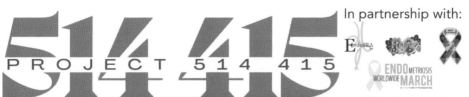

PROJECT 514 415

In partnership with:

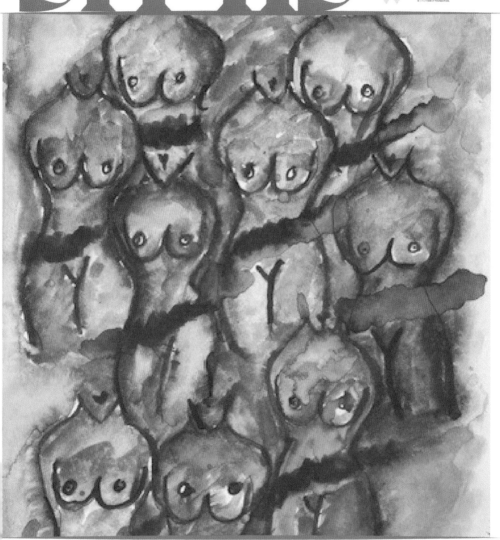

The WHO & NHS states that
1in10 people have endometriosis

www.project 514 415.com
Sharing the Lived Experiences of Endometriosis

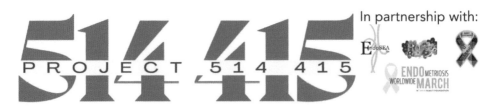

Misconceptions
of Endometriosis

Endometriosis has many misconceptions both within the medical profession and society which not only delays diagnosis, but can result in outdate and / or inappropriate medical treatment and advice. The main misconceptions are:

- Endometriosis is just a painful period that can cause infertility.
- Endometriosis only affects menstruating women.
- The pill, coil, or pregnancy will reduce / slow down / reverse /stop the growth of endometriosis.
- A Hysterectomy or menopause will cure endometriosis.
- Endometriosis is only found in the womb & ovaries (reproductive organs).
- It is too rare for Endometriosis to be found outside of the pelvic cavity.
- Endometriosis only affects women in their 30s who have not had children.

It is vital that these misconceptions are abolished, and that everyone has a factual baseline knowledge of endometriosis.

www.project 514 415.com
Sharing the Lived Experiences of Endometriosis

But all I Hear is Blame

I've come to you with painful periods but all I hear is blame.
You tell me "this pain is what a woman goes through,"
Then you send me on my way.

I've come to you for help but all I hear is blame.
I have been feeling unwell and vomiting,
There are questions if it could be my diet so of course I take the shame.

I've missed days and days of my life but all I hear is blame.
The sickness means I cannot go to university or meet up with friends,
Unable to socialise I lay in bed, wishing the weeks away.

I've come to you for treatment but all I hear is blame.
I tell you I am struggling with other symptoms, related to my bladder and bowel,
It sounds as though it's my fault, as you prescribe tablets that are the same.

I've come to you feeling low but all I hear is blame.
I tell you how my illness has ruined my life,
You spend the appointment speaking over me, telling me your stresses of the working day.

You give me a diagnosis of Endometriosis but all I hear is blame.

I tell you about my condition and ask you questions so I feel sure.

You simply tell me that "doctors know best," and we speak of it no more.

By Clare Gregory

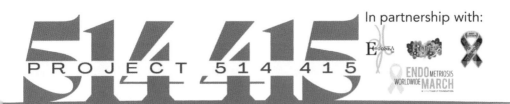

Symptoms of Endometriosis

Although endometriosis symptoms can occur at any time, most symptoms will worsen or start during or before menstruation. Endometriosis is a serious health condition that effects people from all walks of life. If you have symptoms, please seek help.

- Generally feeling unwell during menstruation
- Intense pain in the lower back and pelvis
- Barbed wire sensation around hips/ thighs
- Pain and / or bleeding during or after sex
- Painful bowel movements (sometimes bleeding)
- Pain when urinating
- Nausea / vomiting
- Painful menstruation
- Ovulation pain
- Bloating
- Fatigue
- Unexplained diarrhoea or constipation
- Rib and / or shoulder pain
- Fertility issues

> Endometriosis is an inflammatory condition where endometrium-like tissue (endometriosis lesions) are found in the body which can cause debilitating symptoms & secondary health concerns when not managed.

*Disclaimer please discuss all new, worsening & concerning symptoms with your health care provider

www.project 514 415.com
Sharing the Lived Experiences of Endometriosis

Please Seek Help

If you feel unwell during your days,
know that it is not normal.
Or pain during the ovulation phase,
or during sex or when peeing.

You are a lovely being, and those are signs
that something is not right.
Or when your rib or shoulder hurts
the whole day and even at night.

Or when you are constantly tired,
or when you have a bloated belly,
or you feel like there is a wire
around your thighs or hips.

Or when you have unexplained trips to the bathroom
as your bowels are loose,
or you struggle with constipation,
please choose to seek help.

Or you may struggle with fertility.
Please seek help.
It would be a pity not to see a beautiful baby
coming one day out of you.

By Hana Buchalíková Bujňáková

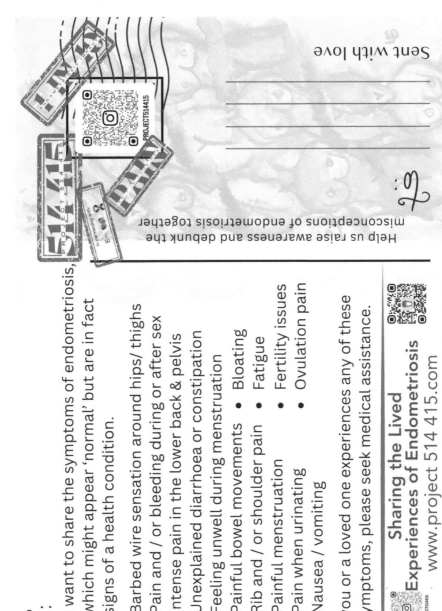

to:

I want to share the symptoms of endometriosis, which might appear 'normal' but are in fact signs of a health condition.

- Barbed wire sensation around hips/ thighs
- Pain and / or bleeding during or after sex
- Intense pain in the lower back & pelvis
- Unexplained diarrhoea or constipation
- Feeling unwell during menstruation
- Painful bowel movements
- Bloating
- Rib and / or shoulder pain
- Fatigue
- Painful menstruation
- Fertility issues
- Pain when urinating
- Ovulation pain
- Nausea / vomiting

If you or a loved one experiences any of these symptoms, please seek medical assistance.

Sharing the Lived Experiences of Endometriosis
www.project 514 415.com

Help us raise awareness and debunk the misconceptions of endometriosis together

to:

Sent with love

116

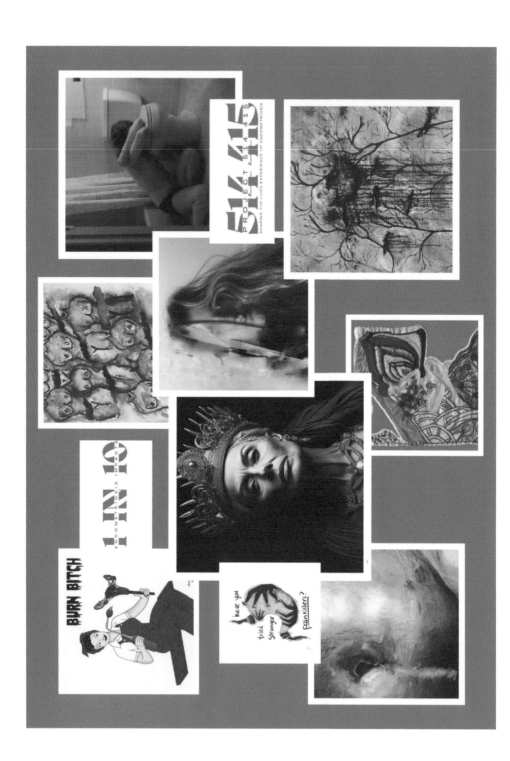

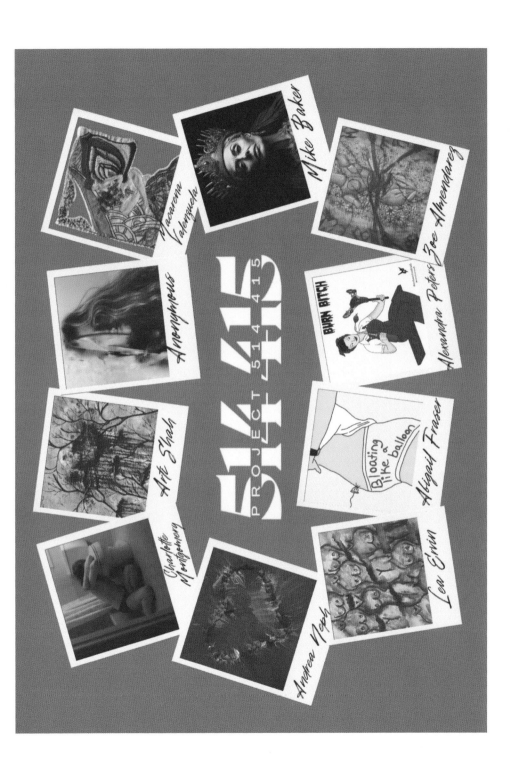

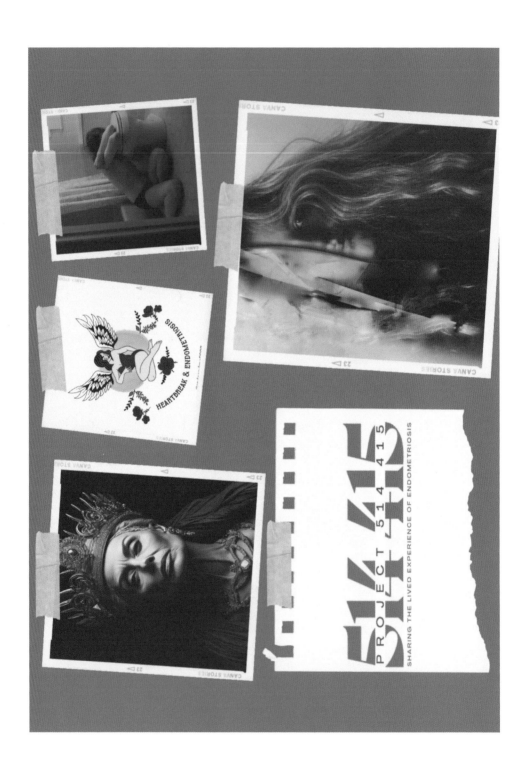

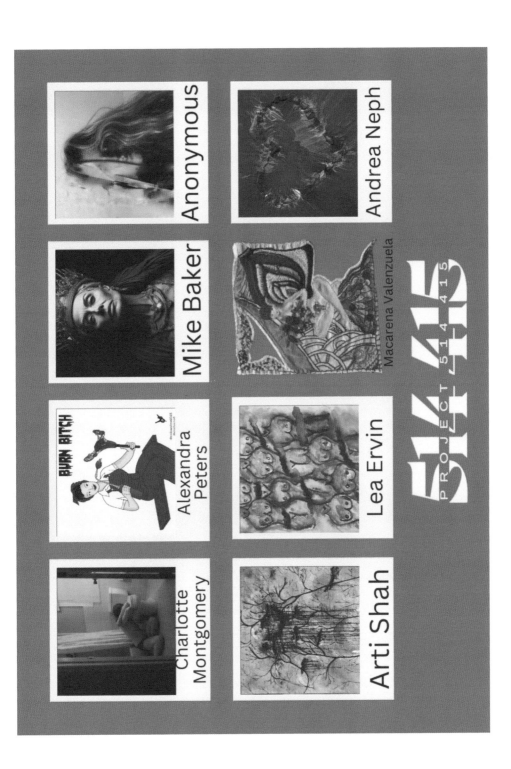

Anonymous

Andrea Neph

Mike Baker

Macarena Valenzuela

BURN BITCH

Alexandra
Peters

Lea Ervin

Charlotte
Montgomery

Arti Shah

PROJECT 514 415
514 415

Thank You

We extend our gratitude to the following organisations for promoting our 2024 endometriosis awareness campaign among their customers and staff. A special thank you to EndoMarch for the opportunity to present Project 514 415 at their endometriosis conference.

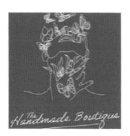

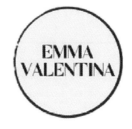

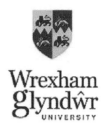

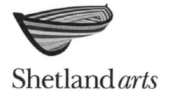

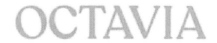

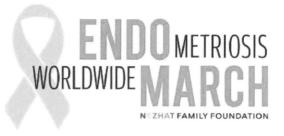

A heartfelt thank you to all the shops, libraries, cafes, community centres, and other businesses who displayed our posters or postcards.

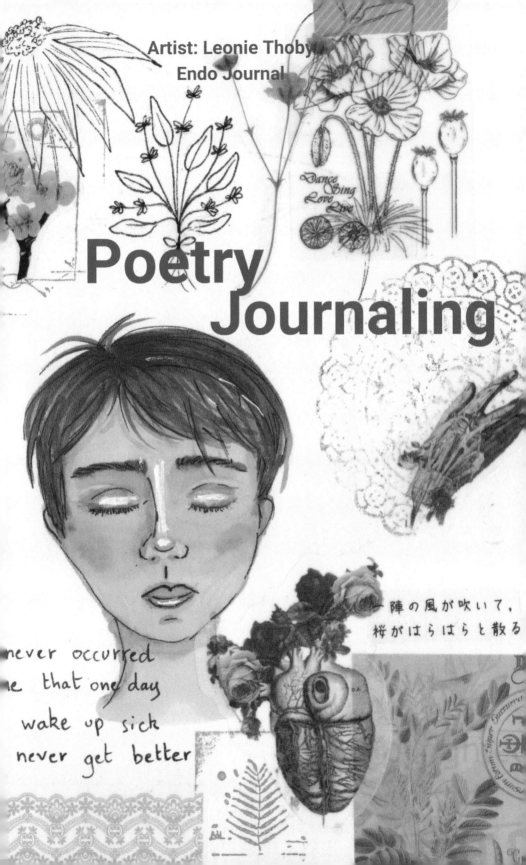

Artist: Leonie Thoby
Endo Journal

Poetry Journaling

never occurred
ie that one day
wake up sick
never get better

一陣の風が吹いて、
桜がはらはらと散る

Mindfulness Activity

Read the question. Use the space below to draw a picture or create a word cloud and write your thoughts.

Question: What does endometriosis mean to you?

Now, re-read through and highlight the words and phrases that captures your attention

Endometriosis Traits

Complete the chart below to identify your experiences with endometriosis and the endometriosis traits that have impacted you.

Negative	Indifferent	Positive

Example of things that you can explore: Symptoms, effects, your thoughts & feelings, the actions towards you, how your character has changed, research, side effects, prior to diagnosis, future, treatment, medication, management etc.

ENDO ART INSPIRATION

Complete the chart below with your thoughts and feelings

Artwork	What is this artwork saying to you? What draws you to it?	How does this artwork make you feel / what emotions?	What textures / patterns / colours do you notice? What does it remind you off?
 Artist: Savannah Dasilva			
 Artist: Carole Thomson			
 Artist: Lea Ervin			

WHAT THEY SAID / DID...

Draw, write or describe a moment you had with your endometriosis experiences.

Most supportive:

The worst thing:

What I wished they would say / do:

Most emotional

The biggest surprise:

Now, re-read through and highlight the words and phrases that captures your attention

Explore one of your endometriosis experiences

The Experience:

Who was there?

What Happened:

1

Where were you?

2

3

When was it?

4

5

How did you feel?

6

Now, re-read through and highlight the words and phrases that captures your attention

4-3-2-1 ENDO-Reflection

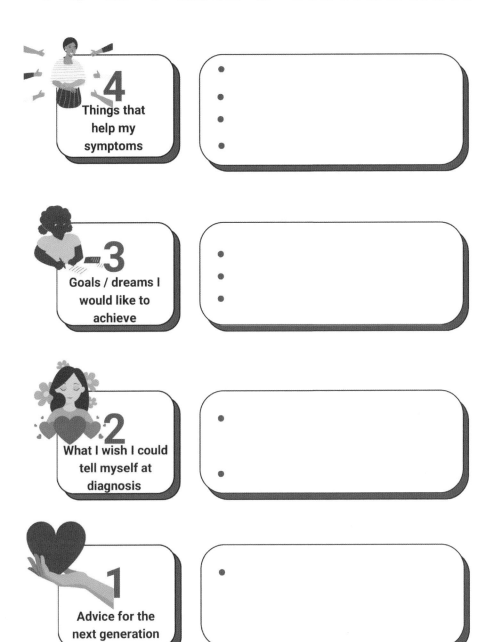

4 Things that help my symptoms

-
-
-
-

3 Goals / dreams I would like to achieve

-
-
-

2 What I wish I could tell myself at diagnosis

-
-

1 Advice for the next generation

-

ENDOMETRIOSIS
ACROSTIC POEM

Instruction: Create an acrostic poem using the letters of the word "ENDOMETRIOSIS" to describe what endometriosis means to you.

E _____

N _____

D _____

O _____

M _____

E _____

T _____

R _____

I _____

O _____

S _____

I _____

S _____

Poetry Practice

For each of the sentences below you will write a new sentence that rhymes with the prior sentence. Try to make it similar in context. The first one is an example.

1. It's never ending, just pending

2. As I whimpered on the floor

3. For countless nights I dreamed

4. You got this

5. The journey of millions

6. To be denied

7. Feeling those close

8. Opinion after opinion

9. I know the feeling

10. I have hope

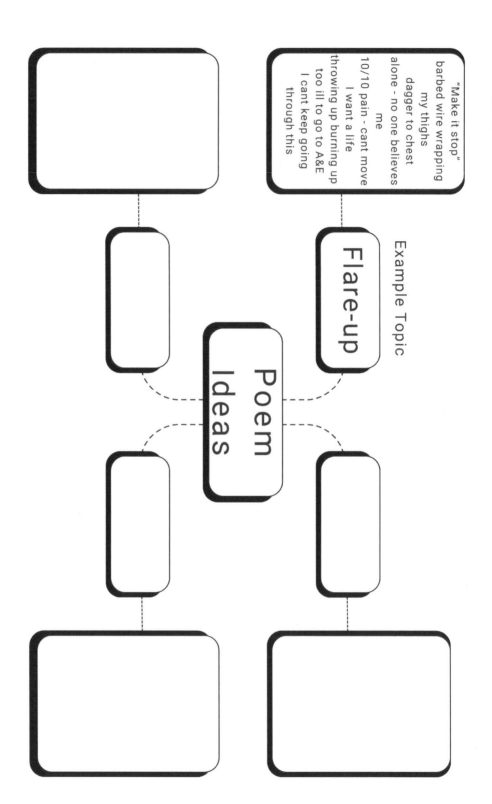

Example Topic

Flare-up

Poem Ideas

"Make it stop"
barbed wire wrapping
my thighs
dagger to chest
alone - no one believes
me
10/10 pain - cant move
I want a life
throwing up burning up
too ill to go to A&E
I cant keep going
through this

131

Poetry Ideas

Use the words and phrases that caught your eye to spark your poetic creation. Here are nine poetry ideas for you to delve into and explore.

Haiku	Palindrome	Acrostic
A haiku has three lines. The first line has five syllables. The second has seven syllables. The third has five syllables.	A poem that reads the same forward or backward. It must be at least 14 lines in total.	Acrostic poems run up and down. You list an item vertically and then write a poem about that item.
Quatrain	**Free Verse**	**Etheree** Consists of 10 lines of 1,2,3,4,5,6,7,8,9,10 syllables. It can be reversed and written as 10,9,8,7,6,5,4,3,2,1.
Quatrains are four line rhyming poems. It must be assigned a rhyme scheme.	An irregular poem that does not follow the rules of traditional poems.	
Sense	**Parts of Speech** Line 1 is an article (a/an/the) and a noun. Line 2 is two adjectives with a conjunction (and/but) between them. Line 3 is two verbs with a conjunction between them. Line 4 is one adverb. Line 5 is one noun (that relates to the noun in the first line.)	**Limerick**
Sense poems appeal to one of the five senses: sight, hearing, touch, smell, or taste. This can rhyme but does not have to.		A limerick is five lines long. Line 1, 2, and 5 rhyme with one another. Lines 3 and 4 rhyme with each other. It is usually funny. The rhyme scheme of a limerick is known as "AABBA."

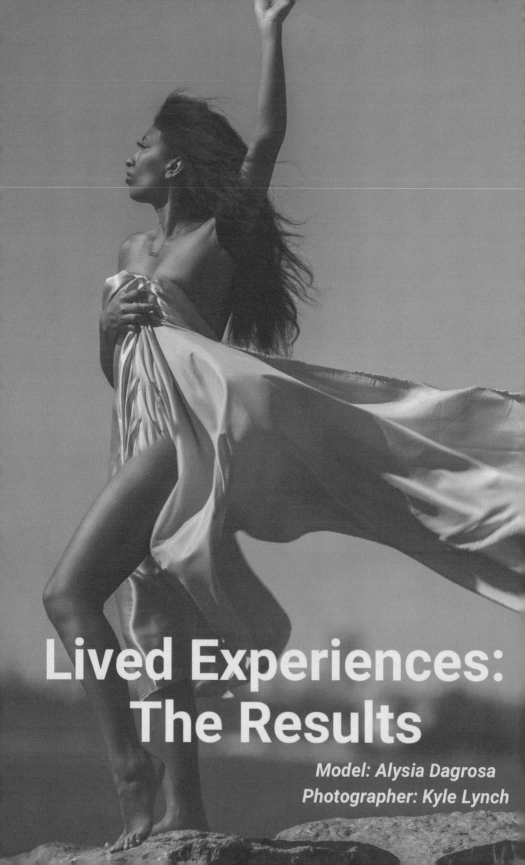

Lived Experiences:
The Results

Model: Alysia Dagrosa
Photographer: Kyle Lynch

The Lived Experience of Endometriosis: Survey Results

We designed a survey to accurately reflect the lived experiences of people living with endometriosis, to address the limitations of existing research, and societal beliefs of endometriosis.

171 individuals participated in our survey, 'The lived experiences of endometriosis'. Unfortunately, 5 individuals had to be excluded as they were awaiting a diagnosis.

Our survey was conducted on Survey Monkey from December 24 to May 25, where we reached out to members of the endometriosis community through social media and on our website. Each closed question enabled all participants to share additional comments freely via a comment box, avoiding limitations from a pre-set dropdown menu and potential biases from Project 514 415. We encouraged participants to have their say by including open ended questions.

We have showcased the data using various methods, including charts, direct quotes from participants, word clouds, and statistical measures like mean, median, and mode whenever applicable.

The Lived Experiences of Endometriosis: Age when endometriosis symptoms started

Individuals partaking in our survey experienced their first onset of endometriosis symptoms between the ages of 8 to 38, with an median age of 23 years (2% of the participants).

Our survey reports that the majority of people experienced endometriosis symptoms at the age of 12 (16% of participants), with the average age being 15 years (15% of the participants).

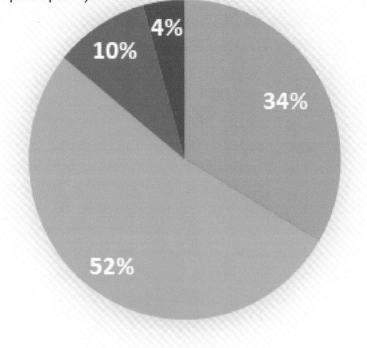

4%

10%

34%

52%

■ <12 years old   ■ 13-19 years old

■ 20-29 years old   ■ >30 years old

The Lived Experiences of Endometriosis:
Age when endometriosis symptoms started
-COMMENTS-

"Severe Symptoms - 36, Significant Symptoms - Early 30s, Possible Symptoms - 17"

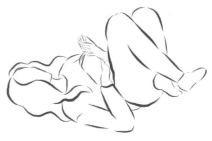

"From 12 but the pain didn't properly start until I was 21"

"16 but it got worse after having my daughter at 22"

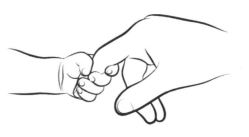

"My symptoms really started to show up at 15"

"Can't remember exactly but in my teens"

The Lived Experiences of Endometriosis:
Age when endometriosis was diagnosed

Individuals partaking in our survey received their endometriosis diagnosis between the ages of 11 to 47, with an median age of 29 years (2% of the participants).

Our survey reports that the majority of people were diagnosed with endometriosis at the age of 26 (8% of participants), with the average age being 28 years (5% of the participants).

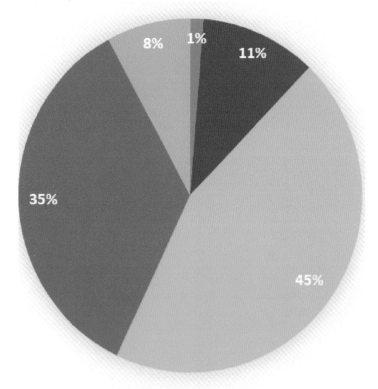

■ <15 years old   ■ 16-19 years old   ■ 20-29 years old

■ 30-39 years old   ■ >40 years old

The Lived Experiences of Endometriosis: Length of time until diagnosed

Individuals partaking in our survey waited between 1- 33 years to receive their endometriosis diagnosis, with a median wait of 15.5 years (5% of the participants waited 15 years, and 5% of the participants waited 16 years).

Our questionnaire reports that the majority of people were diagnosed with endometriosis in 8 years (8% of participants), with the average length of time being 13 years (4% of the participants).

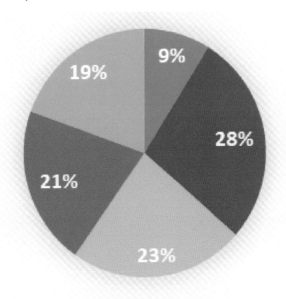

■ <4 years   ■ 5-to-9 years   ■ 10-to-14 years

■ 15-to-19 years ■ >20 years

The Lived Experiences of Endometriosis:
GP visits regarding endometriosis symptoms prior to diagnosis

Participants in our survey reported seeking medical help for their endometriosis symptoms from their general practitioner between 1 and 100+ times before receiving a diagnosis for endometriosis.

We couldn't calculate the Median, Average, or Mode based on the data provided.

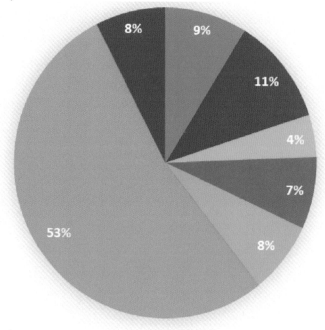

- ■ <4 visits
- ■ 5 to 10 visits
- ■ 11 to 19 visits
- ■ 20 to 29 visits
- ■ > 30 visits
- ■ "Too many" or "Lost count"
- ■ Went stright to a consultant or Gynaecologist

The Lived Experiences of Endometriosis:
GP visits regarding endometriosis symptoms prior to diagnosis
-COMMENTS-

"I was raped by a doctor during my pelvic exam, the first time I tried getting diagnosed"

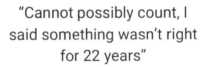

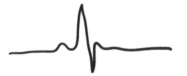

"Cannot possibly count, I said something wasn't right for 22 years"

"I can't even recall, by the time I was 14/15 I had asked my GP for prescription pain medication to cope with the pain ... I was eventually on opiates for the pain...Over 20+ years..."

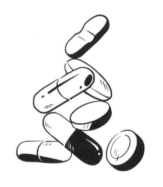

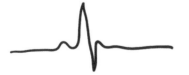

"Every doctor visit from age 16-27"

"At least once every couple months was treated like it's all in your head"

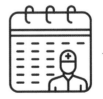

"I didn't really go to them after I was told it was normal pain"

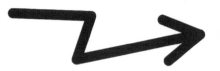

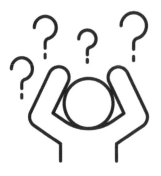

"I went multiple times a year with various symptoms for thirteen years"

"Too many to even count at this point, and I was always dismissed until I found my current doctor. She is a true angel, and I have made sure to tell her!"

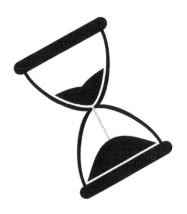

"14 years"

"from the age 11 - 32 zero help or compassion"

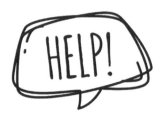

The Lived Experiences of Endometriosis: A&E visits prior to an endometriosis diagnosis

Participants in our survey reported seeking medical help for their endometriosis symptoms from their A&E (ER) between 0 and 100+ times before receiving a diagnosis for endometriosis.

We couldn't calculate the Median, Average, or Mode based on the data provided.

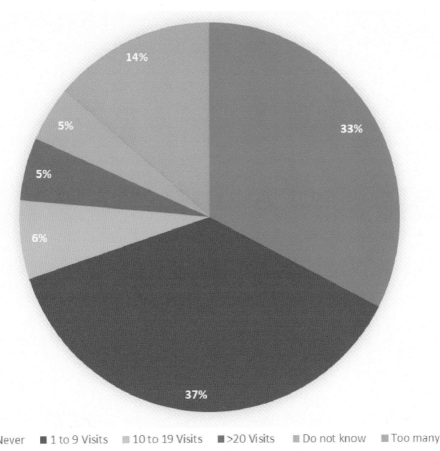

■ Never ■ 1 to 9 Visits ■ 10 to 19 Visits ■ >20 Visits ■ Do not know ■ Too many

The Lived Experiences of Endometriosis:
A&E visits prior to an endometriosis diagnosis
-COMMENTS-

"None, as I tend to gaslight myself since I work in the medical field. I always see so much worse, and always tell myself if I can be here working, it must not be that bad"

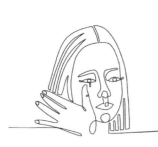

"None, didn't know it was an option. I just cried and suffered at home"

"Never I was too embarrassed it was humiliating"

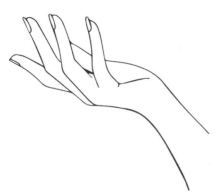

"A handful of times. I tried not to go unless I really had to"

143

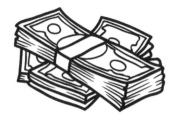

"None due to cost and lack of understanding"

"At least 5 times, with dehydration from severe pain and terrible vomiting/nausea"

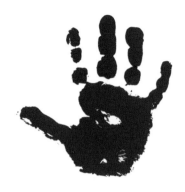

"Too many to count (over 16 years)"

"Countless, over 27 years"

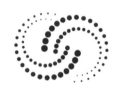

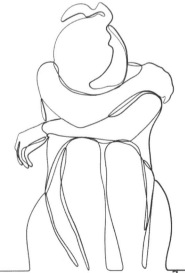

"Once because I don't like going to doctors because of the amount of times I was dismissed, I usually just suffer at home because if not it involves sitting in emergency for hours just to be wrote a prescription"

The Lived Experiences of Endometriosis:
Gynae visits regarding endometriosis symptoms prior to diagnosis

Participants in our survey reported seeking medical help for their endometriosis symptoms from a general gynaecologist between 0 and 30+ times before receiving a diagnosis for endometriosis.

We couldn't calculate the Median, Average, or Mode based on the data provided.

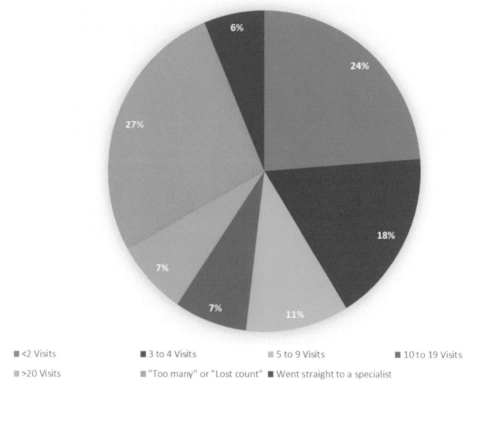

■ <2 Visits   ■ 3 to 4 Visits   ■ 5 to 9 Visits   ■ 10 to 19 Visits

■ >20 Visits   ■ "Too many" or "Lost count"   ■ Went straight to a specialist

The Lived Experiences of Endometriosis:
Gynae visits prior to an endometriosis diagnosis
-COMMENTS-

"Not sure how many, but it was a lot. Since ultrasound and pelvic exams found nothing, I was always 'fine'"

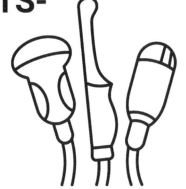

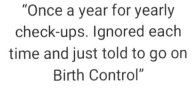

"Once a year for yearly check-ups. Ignored each time and just told to go on Birth Control"

"Too many and many different gynaecologist"

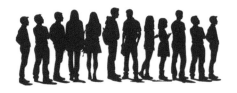

"Way too many to count. I really had to advocate for myself went through numerous until one listened to me"

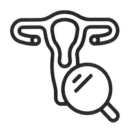

"20+ times... I ran out of doctors to see in my hometown"

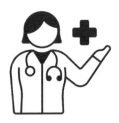

The Lived Experiences of Endometriosis: BSGE gynae or endo specialist visits regarding endometriosis symptoms prior to diagnosis

Participants in our survey reported seeking medical help for their endometriosis symptoms from an endometriosis specialist between 0 and 9+ times before receiving an diagnosis for endometriosis, with an median of 1 visit until diagnosed with endometriosis when seeing an endo specialist (34% of the participants).

Our survey findings indicate that the majority of individuals (34% of participants) were diagnosed by an endo specialist during their initial consultation. Regrettably, 42% of participants never had the opportunity to consult with an endo specialist before their diagnosis.

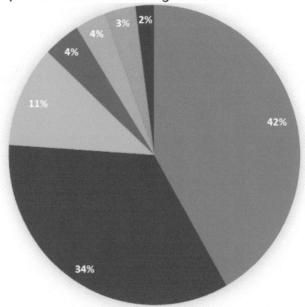

■ Never ■ 1 Visit ■ 2 Visits ■ 3 Visits ■ 4 Visits ■ >5 Visits ■ "Too many" or "Lost count"

The Lived Experiences of Endometriosis:
BSGE gynae or endo specialist visits regarding endometriosis symptoms prior to diagnosis
-COMMENTS-

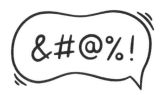

"He wasn't very helpful & was very rude he did not diagnose me"

"Had never heard of Endometriosis until I was diagnosed"

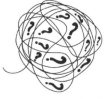

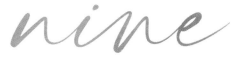

"I saw 9 specialist before getting my diagnosis"

"I saw them as a 2nd opinion after I was diagnosed with stage 4 endometriosis"

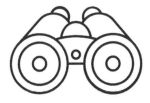

"I wasn't able to see a specialist until two years after my hysterectomy"

"I've never seen one "

The Lived Experiences of Endometriosis: Endometriosis symptoms prior to diagnosis

Participants shared the symptoms they encountered before diagnosis.

The reported symptoms under "Other": Bloating, Infertility/Miscarriage, Prolonged Menstrual Bleeding, Fatigue, Chronic Pain, Neurological Symptoms, Interstitial Cystitis (IC), Urinary Tract Infections (UTIs), Shortness of Breath (SOB), Migraines, Diarrhea, Anemia, Brain Fog, Numbness, and Shooting Pains.

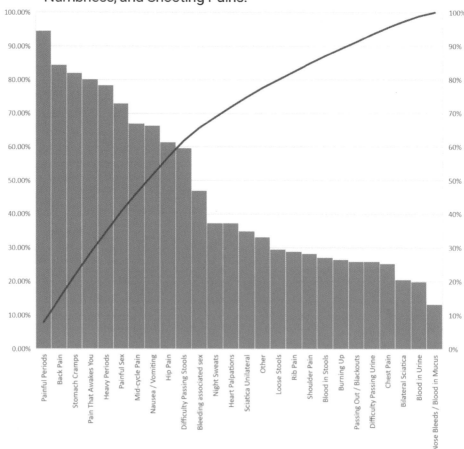

The Lived Experiences of Endometriosis: Endometriosis number of symptoms prior to diagnosis

Participants in our survey reported experiencing between 1 and 25 symptoms prior to diagnosis, with a median of 12.5 symptoms (12 symptoms = 7%, and 13 symptoms = 2% of participants).

Our survey reports that the majority of people experienced 7 endometriosis symptoms prior to diagnosis (10% of participants), with the average amount of symptoms being 12 symptoms (7% of the participants).

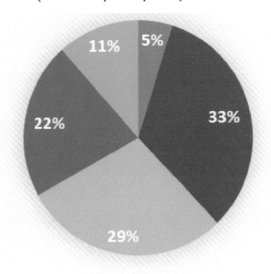

- ■ <4 symptoms
- ■ 5 to 9 symptoms
- ■ 10 to 14 symptoms
- ■ 15 to 19 symptoms
- ■ >20 symptoms

SymptomsPreDiagnosis
ProlongedMenstrualBleeding
BurningSensation
ExtremeTiredness
BloodInStools HormoneImbalance Pain
BloodInUrine PudendalNeuralgia MidCyclePain
PainfulSex Bloating Headaches Migraines
Sciatica UncomfortableOvulation HipPain
Miscarriages RectumPain LightningCrotch
InfertilityCoughingUpBlood Cysts Nausea
BreastPain UTIs Cystitis PMS OvarianCysts
RibPain Diarrhoea Neuralgia Fainting LegPain
AbdominalPain ChronicPain
JointPain Numbness NoAppetite
Vomiting NervePain
BurningPain
PullingSensation Chills PMDD
Exhaustion PinsNeedles Brainfog BlackOuts
ShoulderPain LowGradeFever NoEnergy PassingOut
Fatigue GasPain Anemia PelvicPain
ShootingPainsInterstitialCystitisCramps
BackPain TuggingSensation NightSweats
ImpactedMentalHealth PeriodPain
ChestPains HeavyPeriods
HeartPalpations
UnableToSleepDueToPain

The Lived Experiences of Endometriosis: Endometriosis symptoms misdiagnosed with another medical condition

In our survey, respondents shared receiving 0 to 10 misdiagnoses while dealing with their endometriosis symptoms:

- 31% were misdiagnosed with IBS
- 28% were incorrectly diagnosed with a mental health condition
- 6% were informed that they simply had a cyst.

Unfortunately, we were unable to determine the Median, Mean, or Mode from the available data.

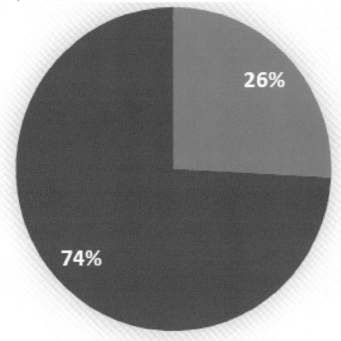

26%

74%

■ Never Misdiagnosed   ■ Misdiagnosed

AdnexalTenderness
HerpesWithNegTest
UnknownAutoimmuneDisorder
CovidVaccineInjuryJustACyst
AttentionSeekingCoccydynia
FibromyalgiaAdrenalInsufficiency
LowPainThresholdChronicMigraines
AnkylosingSpondylitis Costochondritis
SlowTransitBowel**Depressions**
ExtensiveOverlapOfSigmoidLoop
CyclicVomitingSyndrome Hysteria
HemangiomaOnTheLiver Necrosis
ImaginedPain Reflux Hormones **Anemic**
PID **Hormonal IBS** GERD RA **LongCovid**
SpasticColonGallStones Gastritis
Diverticulitis**HerniatedDisc** Arthritis
Asthma GallbladderDiseaseNeg COPD
Anxiety **Hernia UTIs** Anorexia **BiPolar**
PTSD **Appendicitis** GIProblems
FamilialMediterraneanFever
EatingDisorder JustPCOS
ObscuredBowel Dysmenorrhea
ConstipationNormalPeriodPain
SomaticPain Hypochondria
HeavyPeriods LupusNegTest
ChronicFatigue **JustEndometritis**
Hyperchondriac **JustFibroids**
CannabisHyperemesisSyndrome
BarrettsEsophagus**JustAdenomyosis**
EarlyMenopause
AnteVertedUterus

The Lived Experiences of Endometriosis: Endometriosis symptoms misdiagnosed with another medical condition -COMMENTS-

"I was given a diagnosis of bipolar disorder due to the cyclical aspect of my pain, which was affecting my mood and emotions in a way I was unable to see"

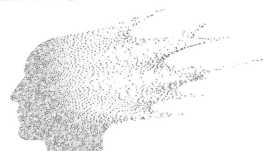

"Anxiety or PTSD related pain, basically told it was because of past trauma"

"Anorexia...driven due to struggling to eat ... I would eat gluten & feel bloated, sick, fatigued, & get stomach cramps.... my periods stop due to not eating, my symptoms went, I felt healthier, I wasn't struggling in pain"

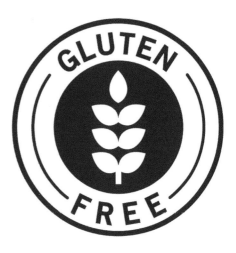

"I felt like a lab rat for many years. My family doctor didn't so much tell me exactly what I had but she kept tossing medication after medication after to me for years"

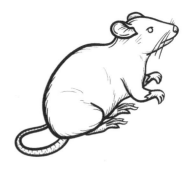

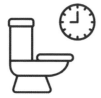

"PIDS, UTI's, constipation, GI issues..... My favourite - it's normal"

"IBS and Period Asthma"

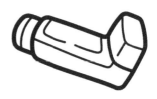

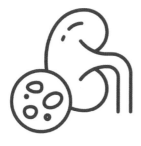

"IBS, Gall Blatter Stones, Kidney Stones, Hiatal Hernia, Hemangioma on the liver and "it's all in your head"

"I had a hysterectomy for unexplained dysmenorrhea at age 37. I asked about endometriosis beforehand but further diagnosis was not explored prior to surgery. Even after that surgery, there was no real explanation for my pain ... I wasn't diagnosed with endo a year later"

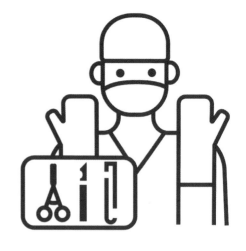

"Yes for year they tried to tell me it was IBS and fibromyalgia"

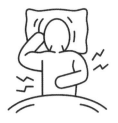

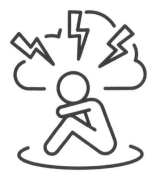

"Anxiety Depression Rumbling appendix 'A tiny cyst that has zero effect on pain or symptoms' Low pain tolerance"

"Severe medical anxiety which was causing me to be a hypochondriac"

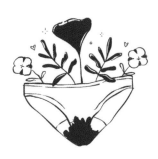

"Early menopause Tight vagina (needed opening more!!) Just period problems"

"IC, fibromyalgia, somatic symptom disorder, narcissism (because i was "obsessed with myself for looking so far into a diagnosis"

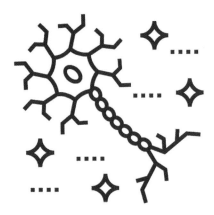

The Lived Experiences of Endometriosis: Incorrect medical treatment given due to misdiagnosis

Our survey participants reported experiencing between 0 and 18 incorrect medical treatments as a result of misdiagnoses while managing their endometriosis symptoms.

We couldn't calculate the Medium, Average, or Mode based on the data provided.

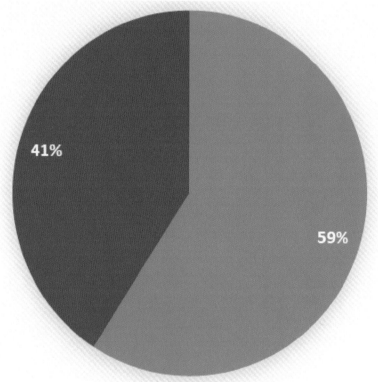

41%

59%

■ Given incorrrect treatment due to misdiagnosis

■ Never given incorrect medical treatment

The Lived Experiences of Endometriosis:
Incorrect medical treatment given due to misdiagnosis
-COMMENTS-

"Emergency appendectomy: no change in symptoms & Birth Control, no change in symptoms"

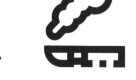

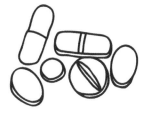

"Anxiety meds SSRI and SNRI (which made me so anxious) Birth control that made me bleed everyday"

"Yes, I was on antibiotics or steroids for almost 6 years straight. I was eating ibuprofen like skittles"

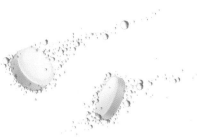

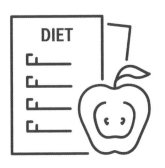

"Low FODMAP diet by GP...wasn't give proper instructions how and was on an elimination diet for approximately 4-5 months resulting in me losing 60lbs and developing a fear of eating"

"18 different types of medication in two years"

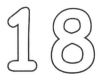

"Counselling Hypnotherapy CBT Many IBS medications All made no difference to my symptoms"

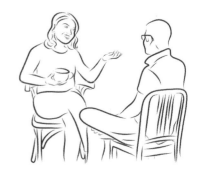

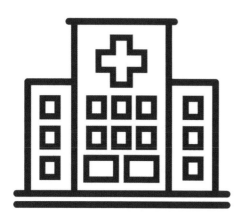

"I was given anti psychotic medication during a flare up that they didn't check interacted with people with endometriosis and it made my flare up worse. I had to stay an extra 2 days hospitalized because of it"

"Told that I should do CBT for pain- told them to pound sand Was sent to do this expensive pain thing that was similar but not CBT for pain (had a pain coach and was psychoeducational modules) after dx of endo and was very invalidating - quit after a month because it really fucked with my ptsd"

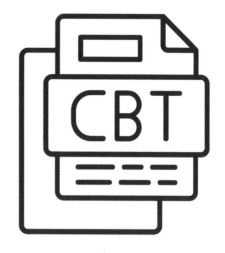

The Lived Experiences of Endometriosis: Medical referrals prior to diagnosis

Our survey respondents mentioned receiving anywhere from 0 to 13 medical referrals while dealing with their endometriosis symptoms. The majority of these referrals were directed towards mental health services (30%), leading to some individuals being evaluated for mental health conditions. Unfortunately, we were unable to determine the Median, Mean, or Mode from the available data.

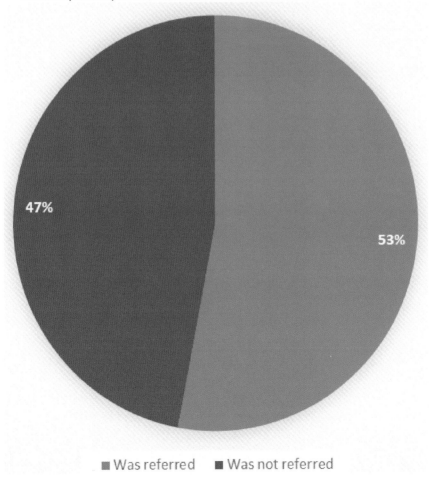

47%

53%

■ Was referred ■ Was not referred

Chiropractor
FunctionalMedicine
InfertilitySpecialist
MassageTherapist
Neurologist
OrthopaedicConsultant   Counsellor
PelvicFloorPhysio Hypnotherapist
Pulmonologist   NoReferral
SexTherapist Osteopath
Cardiologist SocialWorker Haematology
MSKPhysio Therapist Gynea
PainSpecialist WomensGP CBT
Dietician ER Urogynocologist ENT
Colorectal Shaman PainClinic
Rheumatologist Oncologist
Psychiatrist MenopauseReferral
PaediatricEndocrinologist Hepatology
Neuropsychiatrist   Allergist
MentalHealthServices
InternalMedicine
Gastroenterologist
Endocrinologist

The Lived Experiences of Endometriosis: Medical referrals prior to diagnosis
-COMMENTS-

"Cardiologist, gastroenterologist, allergist, ENT, functional medicine, endocrinologist, infertility specialist, OBGYN, therapist. All said I was completely fine and no issues"

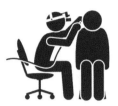

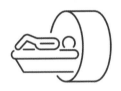

"Orthopaedic consultant who discovered the ovarian cyst by MRI"

"I was denied these referrals"

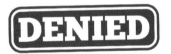

"13 different Drs - everyone passed me to another specialty!"

"Told many times to call a therapist. Very insulting and even though I did the therapy, it continued to get worse"

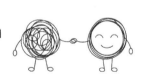

"Psychologist- I enjoyed the therapy, but it didn't change my pain"

The Lived Experiences of Endometriosis: How medical professionals made you feel prior to diagnosis

Among our survey respondents, only 5% described their experience as 'positive' when seeking a diagnosis. In contrast, a significant 89% felt dismissed or overlooked. Even more alarming, 20% admitted to feeling suicidal after their consultation, and 40% reported feeling "Traumatised" following a medical appointment.

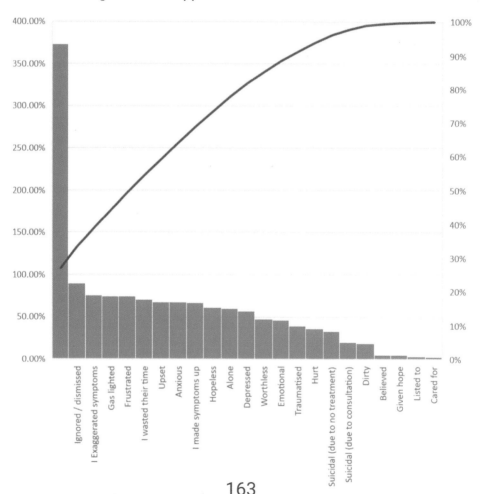

EverythingWasNormal

GivenFalseHope
IMadeSymptomsUp
WastedTheirTime
Dismissed
Mistreatment
PillSeeker
TheyAreNotBothered
TreatedWithNoEmpathy
AnxiousWorthless
Depressed Unworthy
MadeUp
Ignored Scared Pathetic
Alone Informed
Hopeless Weak
Dirty Upset
Unimportant
TreatedEmpathically
Overwhelmed
Neglected
IAmNotTheirProblem
IWasTheProblem
IExaggeratedSymptoms
GasLighted
CaredFor

ABurden
GivenHope
ICouldNotCope
LowMood
Frustrated
Suicidal
Hurt
Clueless
ALier
Poorly
Rude Believed
Traumatised
NoOptions
ListenedTo
Hysterical
Emotional

The Lived Experiences of Endometriosis:
How medical professionals made you feel prior to diagnosis
-COMMENTS-

"I once showed them a picture of the blood I was losing from my bowel and I had one of the consultants tell me I was making it up, they were surprised when I got diagnosed"

"I had a very good experience I was being treated for anal issues with a colorectal surgeon. He asked me a number of questions and he thought it sounded as though I had endometriosis so he referred me to an endo specialist that he worked with. I was then diagnosed swiftly after this"

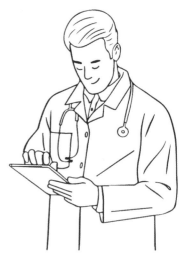

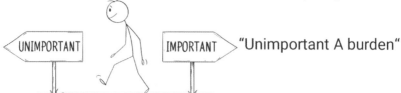

"Unimportant A burden"

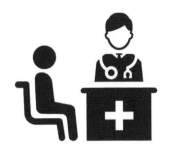

"It's important for me to note that my GP never made me feel like this, he actually took me quite seriously, it was my OB/GYN who made me feel like this"

"I had a constant feeling of dread every time I had to go to hospital or see gynaecology or any doctor about endo. Until one GP who I met just before, they listened to me, supported me and fought with me to get me answers"

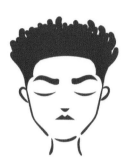

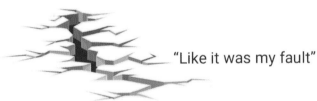

"Like it was my fault"

"Given false hope"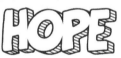

"Hysterical Made up Unworthy Weak Pathetic"

"Neglected "

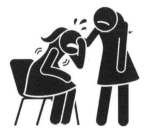

"Things Drs said to me still keep me up at night. OB's should never be treating this FULL BODY disease!!"

The Lived Experiences of Endometriosis: Endometriosis was diagnosed by

Most of the participants in our survey received their diagnosis from a General Gynaecologist.

"My general gynaecologist was the first person who talked to me about endometriosis and immediately sent me to see a specialist"

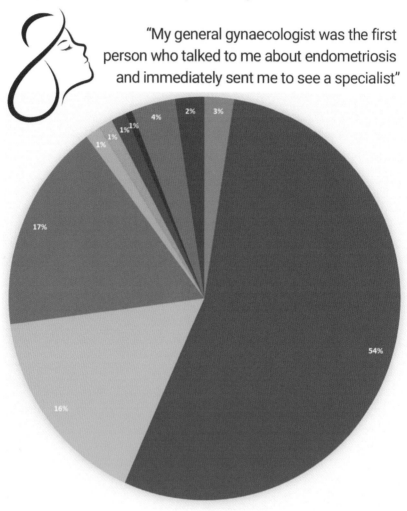

GP

General gynaecologist

BSGE gynaecologist (Endo specialists) Private

BSGE gynaecologist (Endo specialists) NHS / public health

Emergency surgery

Reproductive surgeon

Urogynecologist

Pediatric Gynecologist (US)

Gynecological oncologist

Radiologist

The Lived Experiences of Endometriosis: Endometriosis was diagnosed by -COMMENTS-

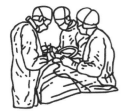

"A gyn diagnosed with ablation in 2019. Excision specialist is my current surgeon"

"Seeking answers for years and visiting many, many doctors, psychiatrist, obgyn and specialists"

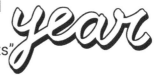

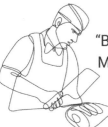

"Both general gyno and endometriosis MIGS gyno which gave me false hope and butchered my insides"

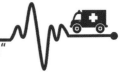

"Emergency surgery after I collapsed"

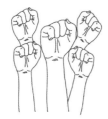

"General gynae to begin with but done nothing about it spent years fighting to get referred to specialists who also confirmed endometriosis"

"I BEGGED an Infertility doctor to do a lap. It was smart because he knew what he was looking at. He did ablation but it was a hot mess"

The Lived Experiences of Endometriosis: Amount of endometriosis surgeries

Participants in our survey have undergone surgeries for endometriosis ranging from 0 to 18 times, with an average of 3 surgeries (18% of respondents). The survey reveals that most individuals had one surgery (34% of participants), with the median number of surgeries being 9.

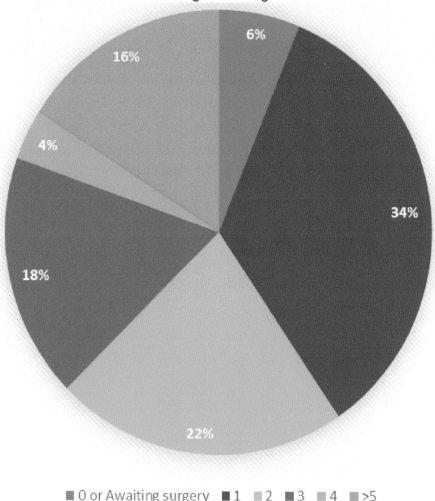

■ 0 or Awaiting surgery ■ 1 ■ 2 ■ 3 ■ 4 ■ >5

The Lived Experiences of Endometriosis: Organs removed following endometriosis surgeries

77 participants (46%) reported having one of more organ removed due to endometriosis.

Other organs listed were: Segment of Vaginal Canal, Artery in Left Glute, Bowel, Small Intestine, Large Intestine Vaginal Septum, Iliac Vessel, and Rectum.

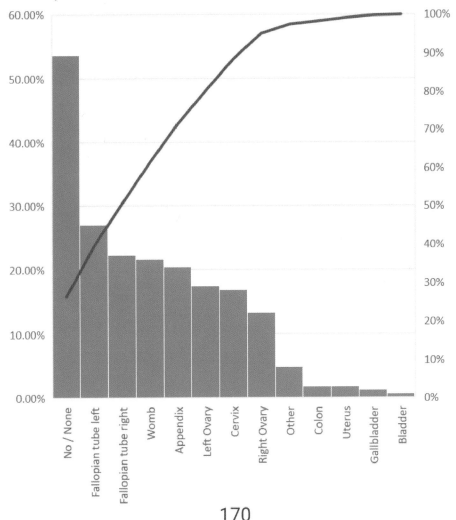

The Lived Experiences of Endometriosis:
Organs removed following endometriosis surgeries
-COMMENTS-

"Failed complete hysterectomy due to adhesions. Only able to remove left ovary"

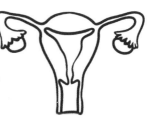

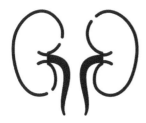

"Seeking I haven't yet but I am waiting for full hysterectomy and possible kidney removal answers for years and visiting many, many doctors, psychiatrist, obgyn and specialists"

"My Left Ureter was cut and re-implanted into a different part of my bladder. I will have hydronephrosis of the left kidney for the rest of my life"

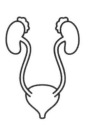

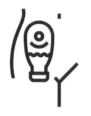

"Bladder relocated and I now have a stoma"

The Lived Experiences of Endometriosis:
Cost of medical treatment due to endometriosis

Our survey respondents reported spending between 0 and £300'000 on endometriosis treatment. The majority of the respondents stated that they have "lost count" or spent "too much" on treatment (25%).

Unfortunately, we were unable to determine the Median, Mean, or Mode from the available data.

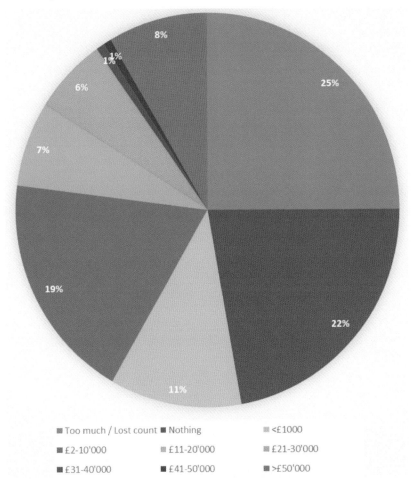

Legend:
- Too much / Lost count
- Nothing
- <£1000
- £2-10'000
- £11-20'000
- £21-30'000
- £31-40'000
- £41-50'000
- >£50'000

The Lived Experiences of Endometriosis: Classification of endometriosis

" 90 survey respondents mentioned receiving multiple classifications, with one respondent even receiving 6 classifications (Grade 4, complex, deep infiltrating, Respiratory, Rectovaginal). Most participants were categorised with deep infiltrating endometriosis.

"I'm concerned my endometriosis has spread beyond my initial diagnosis where it was just around my uterus and ovaries. I worry it's infiltrated my bowels, but no one believes me or will investigate." Classified with G.2 Endometriosis" "

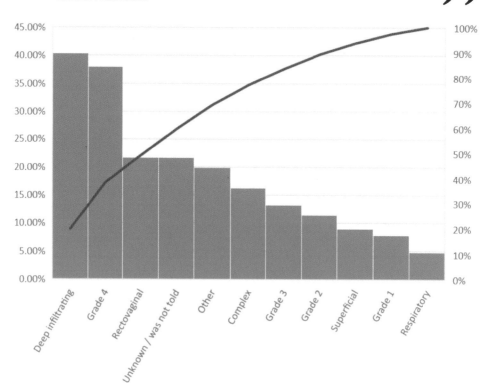

The Lived Experiences of Endometriosis: Where Endometriosis was found

Participants mentioned that endo was found in the the following under 'other': Arteries, Colon, Intestine, Other Nerves, Abdomen Wall, Heart, Intestines, Liver, Other Ligaments, Perineum, Psoas, Veins, Ureters, Vagina, Vessels, and Rectum.

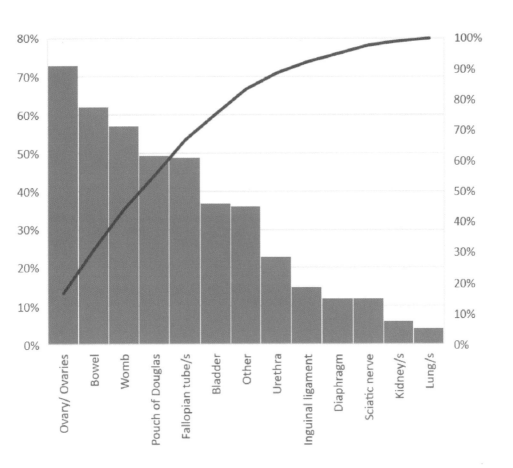

AbdomenWall
Ligaments
VesselsArteries
OvariesNerves
PouchOfDouglas
Diaphragm
LiverKidneyVagina
VeinsUrethraHeart
BladderPsoas
ColonLungsWomb
FallopianTubes
BowelUreters
RectumIntestine
Perineum
Intestines

The Lived Experiences of Endometriosis: Secondary health conditions

Participants mentioned that endo resulted in the following 'Other' medical conditions due to endometriosis: Migraines, Medical PTSD, Chronic Pain, Anemia, Hormonal Lupus, Hormone Imbalance, Metabolic Issues, Compromised Immune System, Food Intolerance, Malnourishment, MSK Symptoms, Prescription Side Effects such as Osteoporosis, Nerve Damage, Surgical Menopause, Other Pelvic Conditions such as Haemorrhagic Ovarian Cysts, Pudendal Neuralgia, and Pelvic Dysfunction.

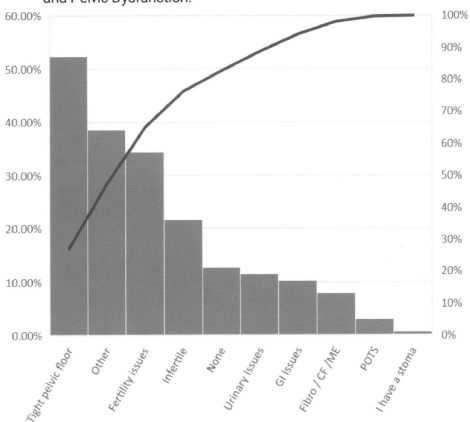

PELVICCONDITIONS
PUDENDALNEURALGIA
GIISSUES
TIGHTPELVICFLOOR
FERTILITYISSUES
GERD STOMA
INTERSTITIALCYSTITIS
BLADDERINCONTINENCE
BOWELINCONTINENCE
URINARYRETENTION ANIMA
FOWLERSSYNDROME
FIBROMYALGIA POTS
CYSTS INFERTILE
CHRONICFATIGUE
URINARYISSUES
PELVICDYSFUNCTION
SURGICALMENOPAUSE

The Lived Experiences of Endometriosis:
Current endometriosis symptoms

Survey participants shared their endometriosis symptoms that they currently encounter. Here are the reported symptoms under "Other": Bloating, Fatigue, Chronic Pain, Neurological Symptoms, Shortness of Breath (SOB), Migraines, Diarrhea, Anemia, Brain Fog, Lightening Crutch, Loss of Mobility, Stabbing Pains, Spotting, Ovulation Pains, Numbness, Shooting Pains, Bowel and Urinary Incontinence.

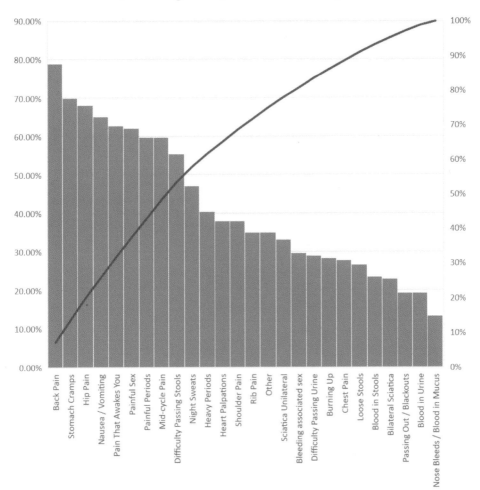

The Lived Experiences of Endometriosis:
Current endometriosis symptoms
-COMMENTS-

"Miserable leg pains, bowel, and urinary incontinence, chronic fatigue, burning sensation in the pelvic, sudden vomiting, intense.., tingling in hands and feet, pins and needles sensations"

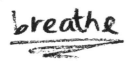

"Winded and can't take a deep breath"

"Brain fog Intense bloating Stabbing pain"

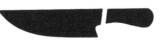

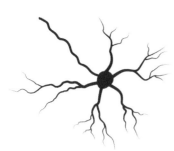

"Nerve pain from my pelvis and lower back all the way down my left leg. So not only sciatica, as this is also on the front, along the femoral nerve. It feels like it starts at the ovary they removed during my first endo-surgery"

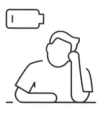

"Exhaustion/tired ALL the time!!!!"

The Lived Experiences of Endometriosis: Amount of endometriosis symptoms experienced

Survey participants reported experiencing 1-25 endometriosis symptoms, with a median of 12.5 symptoms (12 = 4% and 13 = 7%). The majority of participants have 8 cases of endometriosis symptoms (9%), with an average of 11 (6%).

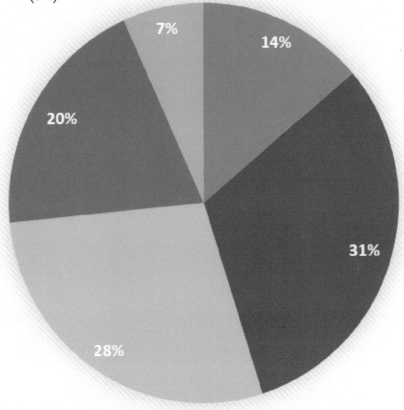

■ <4 symptoms   ■ 5 to 9 symptoms   ■ 10 to 14 symptoms

■ 15 to 19 symptoms   ■ >20 symptoms

The Lived Experiences of Endometriosis: Current MDT

Participants shared the Multidisciplinary Team (MDT) responsible for managing and treating their endometriosis symptoms. Other MDTs included: Acupuncturist, Anaesthesiologist, Cardiologist, Chiropractor, Endocrinologist, Functional Medicine Doctor, Gastroenterologist, Gynaecologic Oncologist, Immunologist, Integrative Medicine, Kinesiologist, Hepatologists, Massage Therapist, MSK Physio, Naturopath, Neurologist, Neurogastroenterology, Nutritionist, Occupational Therapist, Osteopath, Pain Management, Psychiatrist, Rheumatologist, Trauma Therapist, Urogynaecologist, Weight Management.

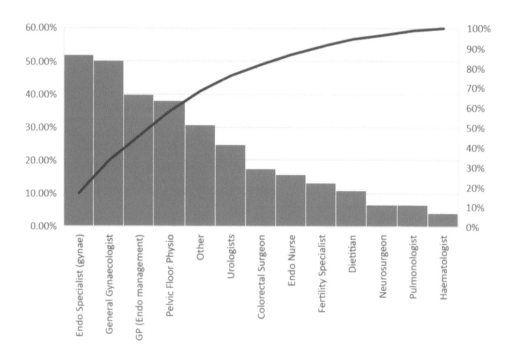

The Lived Experiences of Endometriosis: Amount of MDT

Survey participants reported having 0 - 11 MDT members providing medical treatment for their endometriosis symptoms, with a median of 5.5 symptoms (5 = 10% and 6 = 7%). The majority of participants have 1 MDT (24%), with an average of 3 (13%).
6% of participants do not have a MDT

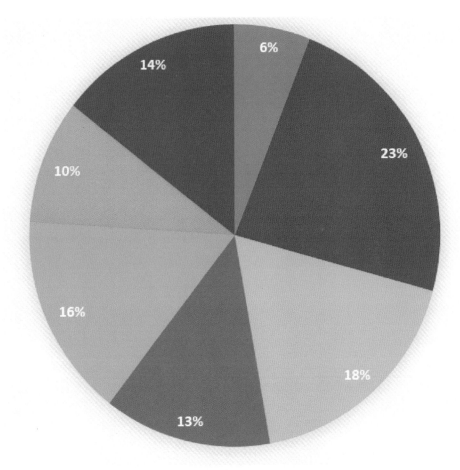

No MDT ■ 1 MDT ■ 2 MDT ■ 3 MDT ■ 4 MDT ■ 5 MDT ■ >6 MDT

Acupuncturist
Gastroenterologist
MassageTherapist
Neurogastroenterology
Rheumatologist Endocrinologist
GeneralGynaecologist Gynaecologic
ColorectalSurgeon MDT
Chiropractor Urologists Urogynaecologist
Naturopath Pelvic Neurosurgeon
Nutritionist Physio PainManagement
EndoNurseGP gynae
Psychiatrist Dietitian Osteopath
Oncologist EndoManagement
Haematologist MSKPhysio
Neurologist FloorTraumaTherapist
FertilitySpecialist Kinesiologist
Pulmonologist Hepatologists
EndoSpecialist Immunologist
WeightManagement Cardiologist
OccupationalTherapist
IntegrativeMedicine
FunctionalMedicineDoctor
Anaesthesiologist

The Lived Experiences of Endometriosis: Current MDT for endometriosis -COMMENTS-

"None, haven't had any support. Use alternative therapies to try and get by"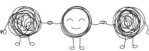

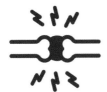 "Waiting to see pain team at UCLH Also see a gastroenterologist"

"Functional medicine doctor helped most also saw endocrinology which wanted me to take metformin for cysts"

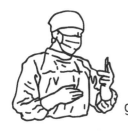 "I'm the US so BSGE doesn't apply. But I saw a gyn who only does surgery and reproductive endocrinology; also see a general gyn who specializes in pelvic pain"

"Trying to get in with a specialist, but no one wants to take my insurance, and paying out of pocket is not possible"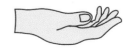

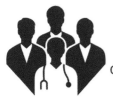 "Under both private and NHS teams - I will have to pay private for treatment due to complicated endo and the NHS being unable to offer excision, also the wait times"

The Lived Experiences of Endometriosis: How GPs made you feel since being diagnosed

After being diagnosed with endometriosis, survey participants revealed that:

- 39% felt that their symptoms / concerns for visit were believed their GP.
- 32% felt they were wasting their GPs' time.
- 33% felt ignored or dismissed.
- 7% experienced suicidal thoughts due to the way their GP treated them.
- 21% stated that their GP understood endometriosis.

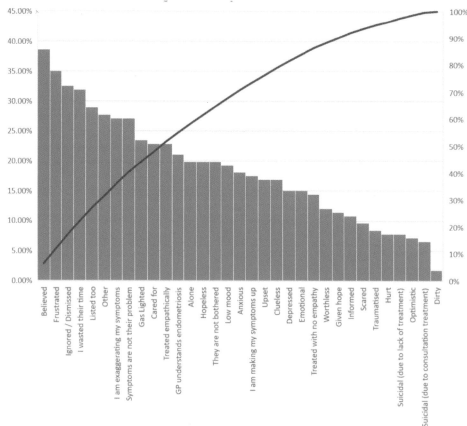

The Lived Experiences of Endometriosis:
How GPs made you feel since being diagnosed
-COMMENTS-

"As though i should be the one with a medical degree from the lies and incorrect information they try to tell me about endo"

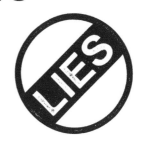

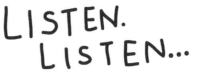

"At 16 after surgery(1st) I was told it was "cured""

"Once I found a caring doctor who listened, I kept him. Been going to him for 12 years now"

LISTEN.
LISTEN...

"Il think my doctors are aware that most of my issues are due to endometriosis but they seem to have the attitude that it's not their problem to make me feel better"

"New GP doesn't deal with my "vagina problems". ..Prior one told me I had no real health conditions and was "impressed your not an opioid addict"

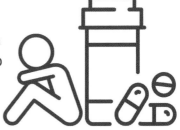

"I gave up on getting help for it after my surgery"

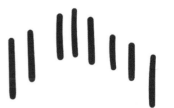

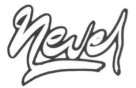 "Never went back to GP and never will"

"GP doesn't understand endo at all but he at least validates my struggle but still thinks I'm being dramatic. He just doesn't know how to assist with treatment options"

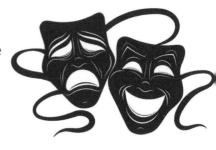

"Literally told me to find a new GP because there is nothing he can do for me until I made a complaint and then I was shown the letter from the previous gynaecologist stating I was 'fixed' no Endo and should get a psychiatric evaluation as it was in my head"

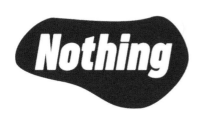

"My GP has always had my back, gyn made me feel dramatic or as if what I experienced was normal"

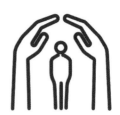

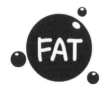 "Fat and treated as a drug seeker "

"My GP is amazing"

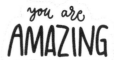

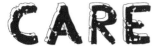 "Caring but unknowledgeable often"

"My GP only believes me now that I got the official diagnosis before that they couldn't care less"

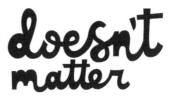

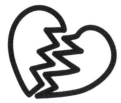 "I don't go back. Medical trauma is hard"

"Unimportant A burden"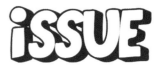

 "Not given range of treatment options. Encouraged to stop breastfeeding to be able to take stronger pain killers"

"As though I am stupid"

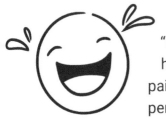 "My GP has laughed at me when i have asked to be admitted due to pain and bloating etc.. She saw me in person and said " oh you are bloated"

The Lived Experiences of Endometriosis:
How MDT made you feel since being diagnosed

After being diagnosed with endometriosis, survey participants revealed that:

- Only 24% of their Endo MDT understood endometriosis.
- 48% felt as though their MDT believed their concerns and symptoms.
- 39% felt as though their MDT listened to and cared about them.

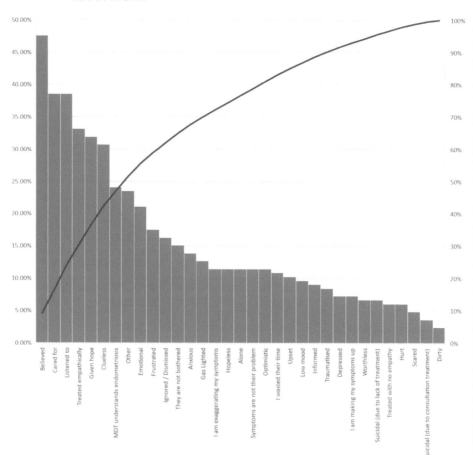

The Lived Experiences of Endometriosis:
How MDT made you feel since being diagnosed
-COMMENTS-

"Like I want to be in pain because I refuse to take hormonal medication. I asked my OBGYN for lidocaine patches for my back pain and she said "if you were treating the endo it wouldn't be an issue"

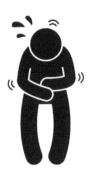

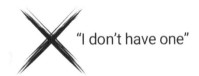 "I don't have one"

"I have seen two one being a General Gynae the other an Endometriosis Specialist. General Gynae made me feel quite stupid like I shouldn't be asking the questions I was asking. My Endometriosis specialist has been wonderful so far and has made me feel heard and talks about best and worst case scenarios clearly"

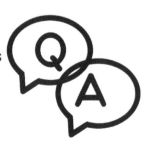

"I was discharged immediately after my diagnostic surgery. No follow up"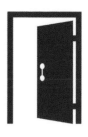

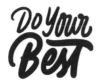 "My gyno tries her best but she is not as educated in endo as I wish she was"

"New surgeon actually understood and was absolutely disgusted with how I was 'left'"

 "Encouraged to rule out other possibilities for causes of remaining / returning symptoms, rightfully so and heard out along the way"

"I don't see any in my country due to having only problems with thoracic endometriosis"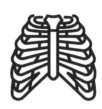

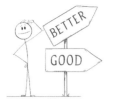 "Overall, I feel I need and deserve better than I've received so far"

" Validated"

"Been really supportive"

 "No care after I was diagnosed. I had to really push for help"

"Abuse of power, no will to correct mistakes "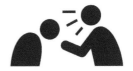

 "My endo specialist is amazing - he is constantly giving me supplements to take, books to read, etc. and reminds me that endo is a full body disease and that everything we do affects how our body responds to endo"

"There is a notable divide between knowledge in NHS and my private team.. My NHS team seem to have outdated knowledge on endo, which is frustrating"

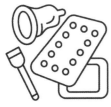 "At this point, my OBGYN tells me they can't help me except to give me birth control.."

The Lived Experiences of Endometriosis: Misconceptions told by MDT

Concerningly, only 19% of our participants were not told any misconceptions by their MDT regarding endometriosis. Surprisingly, 67% were informed that hormonal medication could cure or halt the progression of endometriosis, while 43% were advised to conceive or told that pregnancy was a cure.

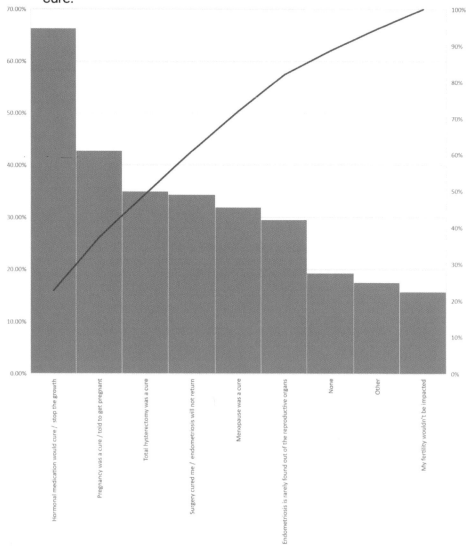

The Lived Experiences of Endometriosis: Misconceptions told by MDT

Survey participants reported being told 0 - 7 misconceptions by their MDT throughout diagnosis or management of their condition, with a median of 3.5 symptoms (3 = 13% and 4 = 12%). The majority of participants have heard 1 misconceptions from their MDT (22%), with an average of 3 (13%).

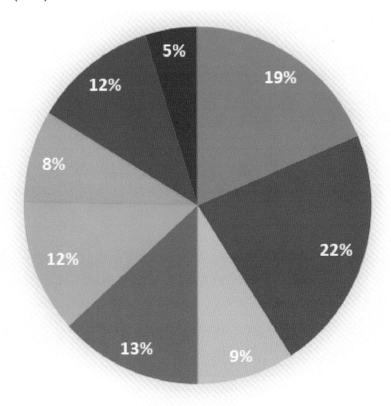

■ None   ■ 1 Misconception   ■ 2 Misconceptions

■ 3 Misconceptions ■ 4 Misconceptions ■ 5 Misconceptions

■ 6 Misconceptions ■ 7 Misconceptions

The Lived Experiences of Endometriosis: Misconceptions told by MDT
-COMMENTS-

"That it can't be that bad since I am so young"

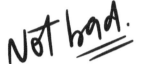 Not bad.

"Each surgeon acted like their surgery would cure my endo"

"Strongly urged to get a hysterectomy because although it wouldn't cure it, it would remove all symptoms even though she knows it's on my bowel and bladder"

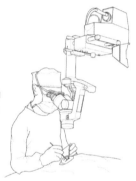

"That endometriosis is the womb lining, that attaches to organs"

"Was also told hormonal medications help keep the endo from returning after surgery. Also was told by a GP that my endo could be cured by diet changes"

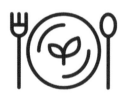

"A variety of incorrect info like try yoga when I had a blocked ureter that made my kidney swell"

The Lived Experiences of Endometriosis: Flare-up symptoms

On average participants experience 9 Flare-up symptoms (13%). With other symptoms being: Contraction-like Cramping, Insomnia, Diarrhoea, Bloating, Pins & Needless, Numbness, Radiating Pain, Vertigo, Night Sweats, Hot Flushes, Indigestion, Gas Pain, Brain Fog, Vision Problems, Breast Swelling, Breast Pains, Deep Vaginal Stabbing Pain, Bladder Pain, Urgency to Urinate, Inability to Empty Bladder, Burning Pain, Can't Walk, Ovary Pain, Full Body Pain, Feel as Though I am Dying, Neuropathic Pain, Muscle Weakness, Immobility, Irritability, and Vomiting.

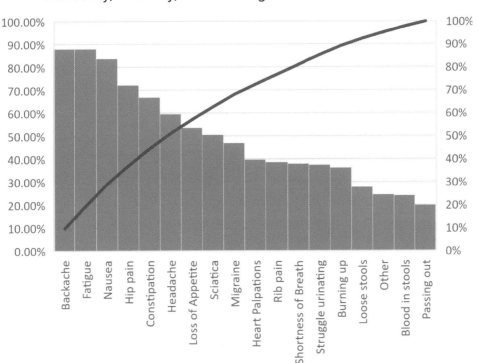

ContractionLikeCramping
DeepVaginalStabbingPain
BladderUrgency
NeuropathicPain
Irritability
Indigestion Sciatica Numbness
ShortnessOfBreath Insomnia
VisionProblems HeartPalpations GasPain
OvaryPain BurningUp Dying HotFlushes
HipPain LooseStools Vomiting Diarrhoea
Vertigo Nausea LossOfAppetite Headache
BrainFog RibPain PassingOut Migraine Bloating
FullBodyPain Constipation CanNotWalk
BreastPain BloodInStools BreastSwelling
BurningPain Fatigue BladderPain
NightSweats Backache RadiatingPain
Immobility
MuscleWeakness
FeelAsThoughIAm
UnableToEmptyBladder
PinsNeedless

197

The Lived Experiences of Endometriosis: Frequency of flare-ups

Survey participants reported experiencing their flare ups daily (14%) to yearly(1%), with the majority of participants experiencing a flare up weekly (24%)

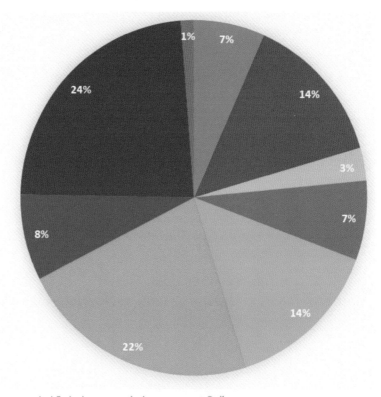

- ■ A few days before my period & during my period
- ■ Period only
- ■ Mid cycle, A few days before my period & during my period
- ■ Other
- ■ Yearly
- ■ Daily
- ■ Mid cycle & during my period
- ■ Monthly
- ■ Weekly

The Lived Experiences of Endometriosis: Frequency of flare-ups -COMMENTS-

"Varies as I've started continuous birth control"

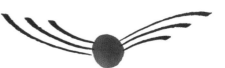

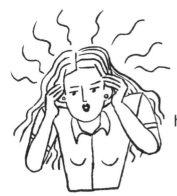

"Post hysterectomy my flare ups happen erratically, can seem to be triggered by stress, and sometimes still cycles out of nowhere. Usually I have a flare up every few months, but not in a cycle I have found yet"

"Sometimes daily"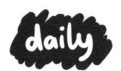

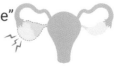

"More like every other month maybe occasional 1-2 day flares here and there. But I've had a complete hysterectomy- I'm technically considered in "remission""

"Ovulation is horrendously painful for me"

"I haven't had a period in over a year due to meds so no clue on timing"

"The severity varies. The first day of bleeding is always the worst though"

"They can come out of the blue for no reason at all"

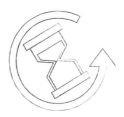

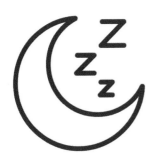

"Honestly, this depends. If I don't get enough sleep a flare up can be triggered. If I eat something I should not it could cause one as well. But definitely being on my period before or after, and during ovulation. Some months is more predictable than others"

"Before expert excision it was daily"

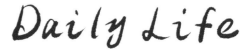

Daily Life

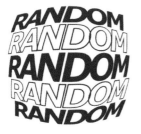

"On the coil so it's random"

The Lived Experiences of Endometriosis: Length of time that a flare-up lasts

Survey participants reported that their flare ups would last between a few hours to months. 7 days, with the majority of participants experiencing a flare up for the duration of 3 days (15%). With other durations being reported as; 14 Days, A Month, 3 Weeks, Comes & Goes, Varies, Months.

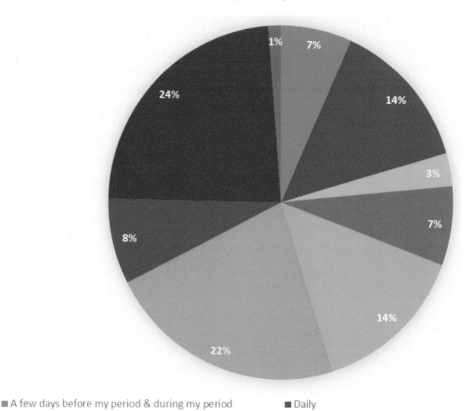

1% 7%
24%
14%
3%
7%
8%
14%
22%

■ A few days before my period & during my period   ■ Daily

■ Period only   ■ Mid cycle & during my period

■ Mid cycle, A few days before my period & during my period ■ Monthly

■ Other   ■ Weekly

■ Yearly

The Lived Experiences of Endometriosis:
Length of time that a flare-up lasts
-COMMENTS-

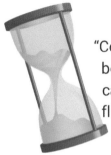

"Completely varies; a bowel flare up can be weeks; during menstruation a flare can be a couple days to a week; other flare ups can last just a couple hours"

"I have been in one continuous flareup for several months -- my complex endo and a bad first surgery caused an inflammatory reaction"

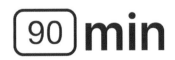

"Hugely varies. Could be a few hours, could be weeks"

"My flare ups last for about half an hour but come back daily, sometimes multiple times a day"

90 min

The Lived Experiences of Endometriosis:
Pain levels during a flare-up

44% of survey participants reported that despite taking pain relief they struggle to eat, sleep, walk and hold a conversation due to their pain levels. Only 3% of participants report that their pain relief manages their pain.

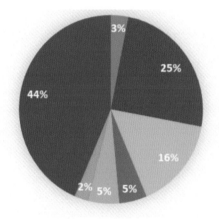

■ Pain is well managed with pain relief

■ In so much pain that I am unable to do anything (I can not eat, sleep, walk, have a conversation, I will be awoken in pain, I will pass out due to the pain) even though I had pain relief

■ In pain but I am able to do ADLs such as eat, sleep, walk, hold a conversation with pain relief

■ In pain but able to do all ADLs & work / house hold duties without pain relief

■ In pain but able to do ADLs & working tasks such as work / house hold duties managed with pain relief

■ In discomfort & able to do all ADLs & work / house hold duties without pain relief

■ In a lot of pain that I struggle to eat, sleep, walk, hold a conversation with pain relief

The Lived Experiences of Endometriosis:
Pending surgeries

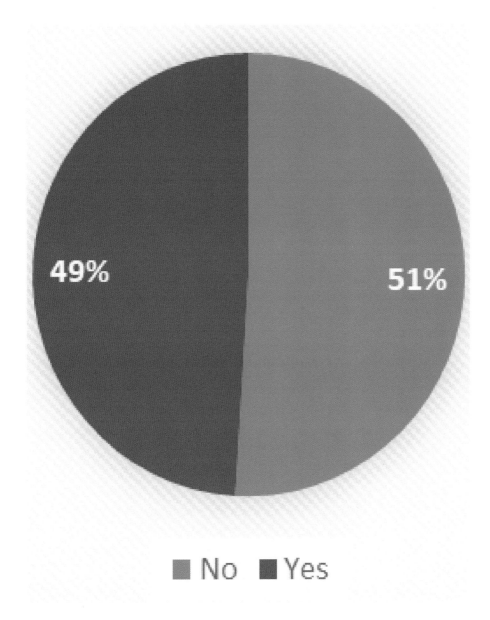

49%

51%

■ No ■ Yes

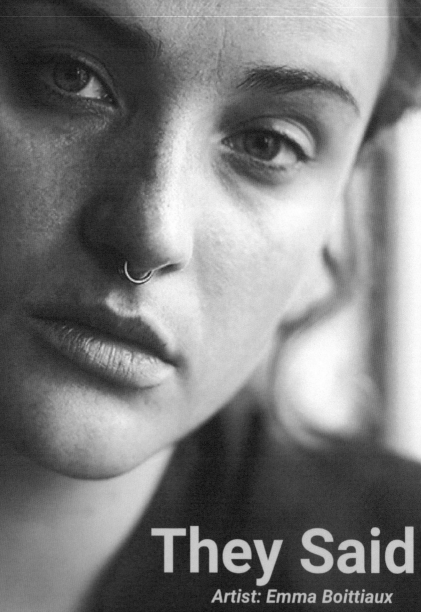

They Said

Artist: Emma Boittiaux
Photographer

What Endometriosis has Taken from Me

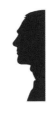

"That's a hard one, but i would say it has taken my identity. Who I was as a person and who I am now, are two different people. And I'll tell you this I miss who I was. Endo had taken who I was, and I can't get it back"

"Everything. I'm 24, have to use a walking stick or crutches to walk. I can barely move. I used to do multiple forms of dance, swim for a swimming club, do gymnastics etc, but endo has slowly robbed me of all of that. I am now existing and often think i can't do this anymore"

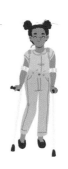

"Education, professional opportunities, belief in myself that I am not making it up that prevents me from seeking any medical attention even when emergency services are warranted for non endo related issues"

"Endometriosis took so much from me, I had to build a new life around it. I would be a different person, a mom, a grandmother, a professional, a traveller, a dancer, an independent person, a healthy body, if I did not have Endometriosis. But what hurts the most, is that I could probably be most of those things if only one person, one doctor had taken me seriously when my symptoms first started at age 10"

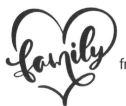
"My entire life: career limitations, loss of financial security, time spent with family, friends, and loved ones, my love for exercising, my mental health, and my identity"

"I have been anemic most of my life so live with fatigue and brain fog .. I feel like I had so much potential that I have never been able to use due to how I feel"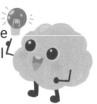

 "My ability to enjoy intimacy, to love having sex with my partner without being worried I am going to be in pain. My confidence"

"My ability to have my own biological children. My spirit, friends, family, my career as a massage therapist, the list goes on"

 "My life that I should be living, not surviving"

"My ability to be spontaneous. Everything has to be planned out more to help with any flare ups that may occur"

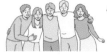 "My ability to work, eat, sleep, hardly functioning, missed out as a teen because of being sick"

"The kindness of my persona I feel like because of the pain is so strong I feel like a raging bitch"

"My career, my independence, my ability to enjoy things without pain"

"My outgoing personality. I used to be so much more fun and active. Now, it feels like I'm always either in a flare up, recovering from a surgery, getting ready for a surgery, or resting my body for a few days after having 1 normal day"

"Time with family and friends. Being able to go out/on holiday without worrying about pain/flare ups. Confidence"

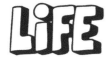

"Quality of life. Now it's about symptom management and coping"

"The chance to have my own birth children, wasted time and money on IVF"

"Everything I've lost a marriage I've lost a baby and I've lost me I don't know who I am anymore"

"Education. Employment. Life. Adventures"

"Everything. My dignity, my health, the ability to sleep, to smile, to laugh. It's taken me!"

Advice to Medical Professionals to Improve a Patients Experience During Diagnosis

"Your words and treatment of your patients ... esp teenagers / young adults, have a life time effect.... I do not trust medical professionals and have trust issues in sexual relationships due to the amount of STI tests I was made to have / being accused of having a STI. I now panic that I will get a STI or that my partner will cheat and give me a STI, even if they have been tested"

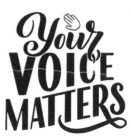

"Listen to what your patients are telling you! They are experts about their body, so even if you don't fully understand what they are saying, ask questions so you can. Please do not dismiss them. This can cause great trauma and lead to altered mental states that we are already struggling with because of the pain"

"There needs to be more training given to staff for a better understanding of what endometriosis is. 20 minutes in med school is not nearly enough for the hundreds of women/girls out there suffering. Rather then dismissing us, hear us, support us and try and put yourself in our shoes before sending us off with just another bad period. We just want to be heard, believed."

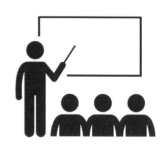

"Believe their pain even if nothing shows on ultra sound / test that it still has to be coming from somewhere physically"

Believe

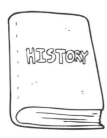

"Listen to your patients. Take the time to understand the clinical history that is in front of you and never, ever forget that you may have learned a lot about the condition and the human body, buy it is the life, the everyday life of your patient you are talking about"

"Just to learn to listen to their patients because sometimes their patients know exactly what they're talking about and probably no more than the doctor but since the doctor has a degree or a PhD doesn't mean that they should just Gaslight us and shut us out and not listen"

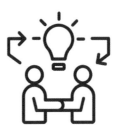

"Don't blame mental health or trauma for everything they are experiencing"

"Give people who don't want children to have proper medical care"

"When a teenager complains of digestive symptoms consider Endo"

"Ask how the pain feels because not every pain feels as similar"

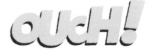

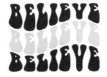

"Don't dismiss concerns around periods, concerning levels of discomfort and pain during menstruation should be taken seriously. It isn't normal"

"Listen to patients and advise them on the basis of belief. Understand that the patient does not know what is going on. Look at all of the symptoms in the round. Ask questions to draw out symptoms that the patient may have normalised"

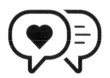

"To be more understanding Listen to the patient first Explain things more or better I didn't really understand endo until after my diagnosis & 3rd time admitted to hospital"

"Endometriosis needs its own specialty! Also more education and better ACOG standards for insurance"

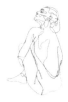

"Listen to your patient. Stop linking the pain to the period. It's not a period disease, it's a full body disease. Bad periods are just 1 of the many symptoms, not the entire disease"

"I don't just have to have a painful sex life or period to be experiencing the pain that Endo causes"

"To believe my pain and to never have OBs treat a full body disease when all they look at is one small section of where Endo is or could be"

"If you don't know much about the condition, be honest. Don't try to pass off incorrect information as the truth. Also, if i say it hurts, it really hurts and i'm trying to get some help!"

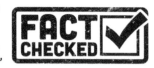

"Don't rate my pain on the results of an ultrasound"

"Stay current on endometriosis instead of using the same outdated information"

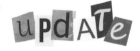

Advice to Medical Professionals to Improve a Patients Experience When Managing or Treating Symptoms

"Have a little bit more empathy when dealing with patients who have endometriosis. We don't ask to have it and we certainly don't exaggerate our symptoms. Try and have a better and clearer understanding of the condition and think before you speak, most girls/women are vulnerable with this condition as it's a hard condition to process"

"Communication of all findings needs to be thorough to enable us to research our health independent of their care"

"Insurance hoops and hospital costs are preventing millions of people from getting treated. Please streamline a path to diagnosis."

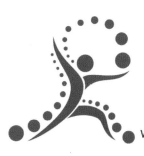

"I just wish medical professionals were better at recognizing whether they are actually skilled enough to be called an Endo specialists. I dealt with at least three doctors, surgeons and physical therapists who claimed expertise but were operating on basic misinformation"

"To work with their patient. Ask them what they want to do. These patients have done their own research, they know the meds and treatments that are available, so ask them what meds they want to try. If they ask for surgery, give it to them. If they ask for a certain test, give it to them. No one is going to the doctor for fun, no one is trying to get billed for fun, they are there looking for help so they can live their life comfortably, so listen to what they need and work with them"

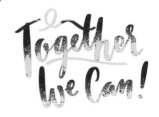

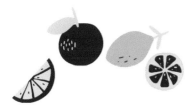

"More information on how to manage daily not just given hormonal treatment / pain relief and surgery. We need a plan on how to manage a diet, pain management, physio etc"

"Endometriosis is a cureless, chronic and painful disease. You should think of long term side effects of treatments as well as life quality enhance options"

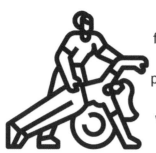

"After my last operation in Germany, I was sent to a rehabilitation centre where I was followed with physiotherapy, massages and instructed for three weeks on nutrition, physical and psychological therapies, how to create a daily routine; where I found other women with the same condition as me and where I felt I was not alone. This would be great if it were available to everyone"

213

"Suggest other ways to help manage living with the disease going forward such as, seeing a Pelvic floor therapist, emotional counselling"

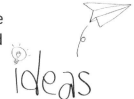

ideas

STORY of MY LIFE

"Please discuss with us that this is a lifelong disease, and not a one and done surgery. We will have repercussions of this disease in every system of our body"

"That there should be some support after stage four surgery. I was discharged there was no medical support"

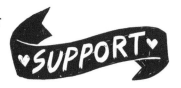

SUPPORT

Help me
Help

"Help me treat the pain and don't make me feel like I'm bringing it on myself by not taking hormonal drugs"

"Do your own research on the possible treatments for specific patients in the areas they have endometriosis: ie don't suggest intrauterine endometriosis treatments for someone struggling with it in their bowels"

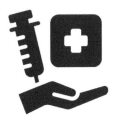

"Don't force treatments patients aren't benefitting from or comfortable with. Acknowledge complications caused by treatments"

"The suggestion of getting pregnant to stave off the endometriomal tissue growing for a time is really problematic. Having a baby should never be suggested as treatment"

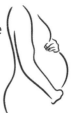

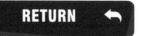

"Endo can still come back even if you are a great surgeon. I know my body best"

"Follow up with patients, leaving them isolated with chronic pain is unacceptable"

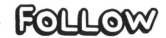

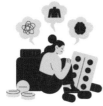

"Toradol is not a narcotic. And even if it was, please don't act like I'm a drug addict for asking for it with a 25cm incision in my abdomen"

"Stop forcing "treatments" on patients who feel uncomfortable taking them and actually give informed consent so patients can make the best choices for them. Also look at this condition as a whole body disease"

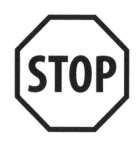

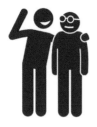

"Be reassuring whilst also remaining realistic. We know there isn't a cure but we need support from the people who have the power to literally save our lives"

The Dr Said...

He threw, threw my pain journal across the room

At your age the only real symptoms We are worried about is infertility. You don't even have a partner why are you so concerned?

I'm not here to give you a science lesson. You go fly around the world for a. Second opinion then come back to me

What you are going through is normal for some women

Why did you come to the ER to be told to take a Tylenol?

Your pain is probably karma caused by doing bad things in a past life

You're just fat. Lose weight you'll be fine

More sex will make the pain go away

Learn to deal with it

Endo isn't even that bad

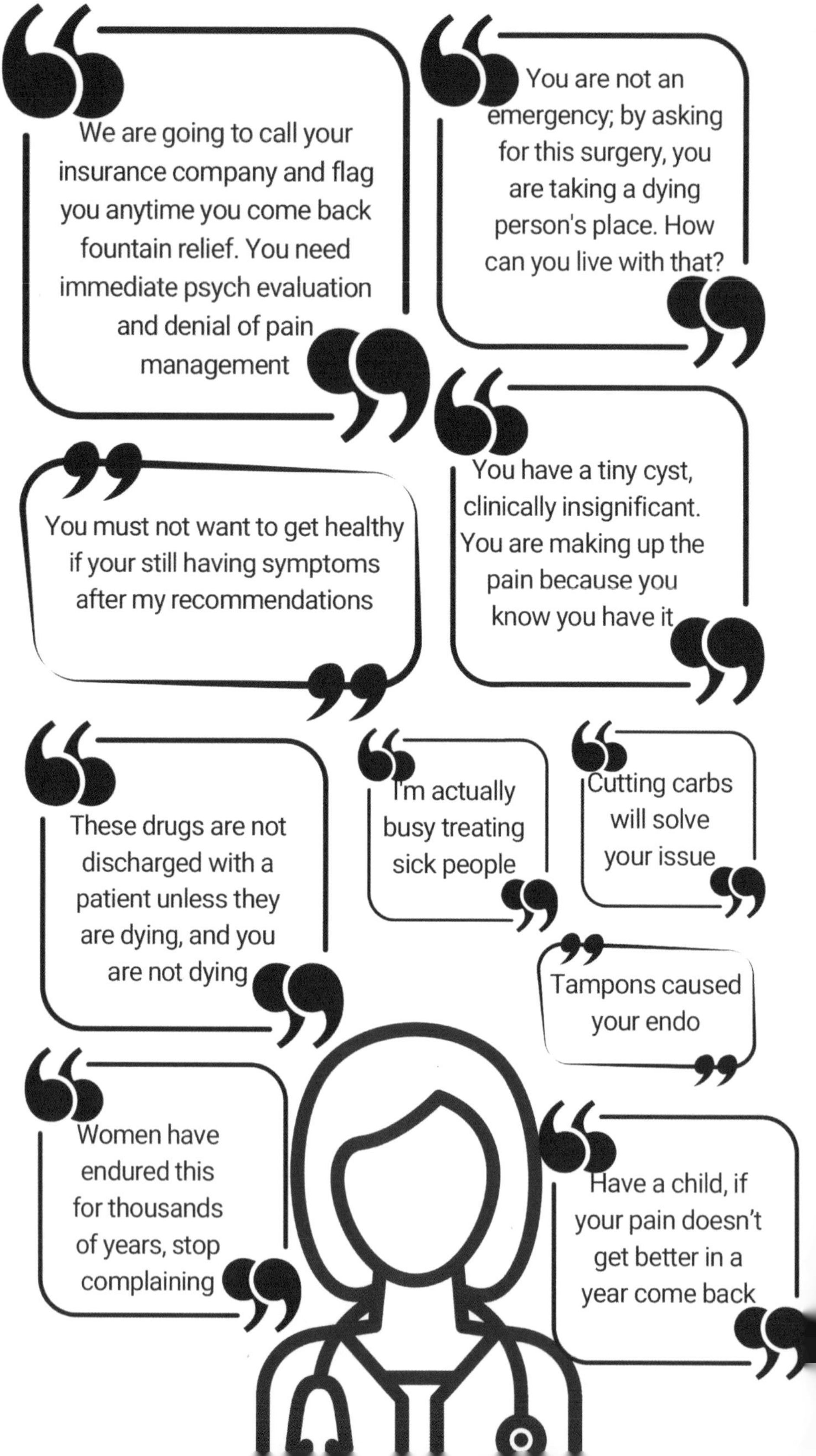
We are going to call your insurance company and flag you anytime you come back fountain relief. You need immediate psych evaluation and denial of pain management
You are not an emergency; by asking for this surgery, you are taking a dying person's place. How can you live with that?
You must not want to get healthy if your still having symptoms after my recommendations
You have a tiny cyst, clinically insignificant. You are making up the pain because you know you have it
These drugs are not discharged with a patient unless they are dying, and you are not dying
I'm actually busy treating sick people
Cutting carbs will solve your issue
Tampons caused your endo
Women have endured this for thousands of years, stop complaining
Have a child, if your pain doesn't get better in a year come back

What Everyone Should Know About Endometriosis

"The seriousness of it. When I was first referred to gynae I never even realised how bad it could be. The people in my life, bless, try their best but I just don't feel connected to anyone about it. It's such an isolating thing to go through and there is no way out, and I'm constantly worrying about the progression and what that means for my future"

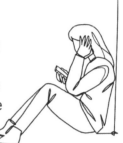

"It impacts your whole life! Relationships Plans / Days out Work / Employment / Studies Mental Health Physical health Well-being Finical stability Sex life / Intimacy Future plans Dreams Holidays Travel (try driving on the motorway, when you all of a sudden you get a flare up hours from home.) Family / family plans"

"That it is very painful so much you think you are dying. To validate that pain and not gaslight you. To understand that one day you can be fine but the next awful. Not to judge someone based on this. That despite the pain some of us just battle on through and do fun things regardless it does not mean the pain is any less it just means that we've learnt to live with it."

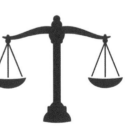

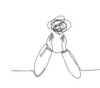

"It's so much more than just a bad period or reproductive disease it's a full body disease negatively impacting your life in every aspect with devastation , ambiguous loss & disenfranchised grief"

"Is a serious debilitating condition for those symptomatic with pain that it destroys the quality of life and time of the patient. They need to be believed when it's not just a simple dysmenorrhoea"

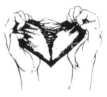

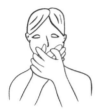

"How painful it is and what we are living with daily. I wish it were acknowledged as a disability without having to prove it. The weight of the trauma of living with it in silence for years because we aren't heard or taken seriously"

"When you don't know what's happening to your body, it's terrifying. More information taught generally could ease this feeling - the first time it happened, I felt like I was giving birth for hours (I wasn't). The pain is horrendous"

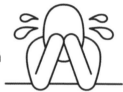

"It's a systemic inflammatory disease. And inflammation can be very painful and damaging to organs and tissue over time"

"It's very very similar to cancer and it IS deadly. Hundreds of people die because of endometriosis every single year. Yet for some reason it's seen as a non-fatal disease"

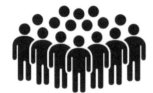

"That it's wayyyyyyy more common- at least if not more than 1 in every women (and even some men!)- and needs desperately to become an international research priority"

"The pain or flare up can come on very sudden and you have no way of knowing how your day will be"

"That it's real and a friend cancelling plans or colleague calling in sick isn't swinging the lead"

 "That is a whole-body disease - We need to stop associating it with only reproductive issues"

"The level of pain being so severe and how often it occurs. That symptoms can vary day to day. That we are not lazy when we need to rest"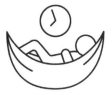

 "Endo is not just a woman's illness"

"How much it can effect someone mentally not just physically"

 "It's more than a bad period and it affects everyone differently"

"How painful and tiring and debilitating the condition is"

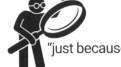 "just because you can't see it doesn't mean it doesn't hurt"

"It can grow back anytime and anywhere. It's like a cancer"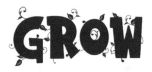

Advice for the Next Generation of People with Endometriosis

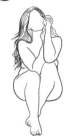

"If something feels wrong it most likely is listen to your body. Even if others won't listen to you keep pushing until you find someone who will! We know our bodies better than anyone else. We know what's normal and abnormal for us!"

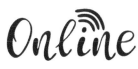

"Go online - you will get more information and community from Facebook groups and social media accounts. then from anywhere else. And you will need to do a decent amount of research in order to be able to seek proper treatment and advocate for yourself"

"Always advocate for yourself. Fight for your body and never let anybody tell you otherwise. It is your body and the only person who knows your body better than anybody is YOU. Don't be afraid to speak up if something isn't right"

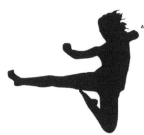

"Fight for yourself. Change doctors if you don't feel one is listening to you. Always go with your gut. Doctors are not all knowing and many times will give you false information than admitting they need to do research"

"Your pain is valid and that validation doesn't depend on affirmation by someone with a medical degree. Doctors make mistakes too"

"Fight, fight and fight some more. You are your best advocate until something in system changes. Have your friends, family and the community to support you also"

"Breath! Get a good heating pad! It's okay to tell others to please stop, if you're getting overwhelmed"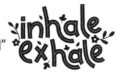

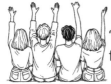
"Advocate for yourself and bring a family member or friend they seem to care more if you are not alone"

"Fight. Because your life depends on it"

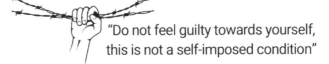
"Do not feel guilty towards yourself, this is not a self-imposed condition"

"The level of pain doesn't always correlate to the severity of endometriosis"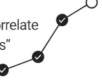

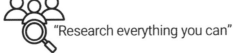
"Research everything you can"

"You might think your symptoms aren't a problem and that this is just life - especially if the other women in your family had similar symptoms. Just because the pain might be normal for you doesn't mean you can't get treatment"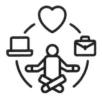

"From my own personal experience, I would tell the next generation to listen to your body and not to see it as an enemy despite all the pain and suffering. Your body is letting you know something is wrong and despite what the doctors say, you are not crazy. Build a good relationship with your body from a point of care and don't see your uterus or periods as the enemy. Women are taught to see their bodies in a very negative sense and it creates a disconnect. The best way to try to navigate this is to build that connection back with your body and do whatever you must to advocate for yourself and the body you're in"

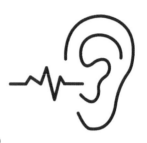

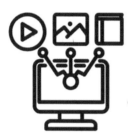

"Always advocate yourself and NEVER be afraid to challenge a doctor or any other medical professional. You know your body better than ANYONE. There are resources out there to help find the proper care, but it's not going to be your local OB/GYN"

"You're not crazy. Your pain is real. Keep fighting and seeking help until your find it. Your body is not against you—it's letting you know that something is not right. Your body will be so glad you didn't give up searching for help"

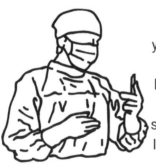

"Don't give up. It might not get better but once you find a doctor willing to work with you keep them. When I finally found a doctor who believed me, he said, "it's not pcos. I'd bet my whole career that it's endometriosis. You need to find a doctor who can do the surgery, but it's not me. I wouldn't know what I'm looking at." - that was the most honesty I ever got out of a doctor"

"Find your voice through research and talking to others in support groups and then advocate for yourself like you life depended on it because it does. Interview doctors for your care team, NOT the other way around. Don't let healthcare workers make you feel like less than or weak or unworthy"

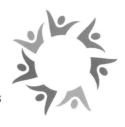

Don't GIVE UP! "Don't give in and have hope, things are slowly changing"

"Don't let it swallow you up. All is not lost. There are so many people in the same boat. You are not alone"

Contributors

Abigail Fraser

Aimee Gill

Aine Drummond

Alexandra Peters

Alice Brunello Luise

Alysia J. Dagrosa

Andrea Neph

Anonymous

Antje Bothin

Arti Shah

Ashlee Britt Rollins

Beth Cooper

Cameron Hardesty

Carole Thomson

Cassandra Nordal

Charley Cutter

Charlotte Montgomery

Chelsea BreeAnn Hardesty

Christine

Claire Chapman

Clare Gregory

Deneika Klynnyk

Donna Jardine

Emma Boittiaux

Emma Gill

Frosty Knoll

Gazelle Pezeshkmehr

Gemma Starvis

Georgina Moon

Hana Buchalíková Bujňáková

Helen Grant

Ine-Sophie J. Berglund

Iness Rychlik

Jessie Jing
Joy Getliffe
Kay Ritchie
Kirsty Clarke
Lea Ervin
Leona McKenzie
Leonie Thoby
Liz Van Ingen
Lorna Merrow
Macarena Valenzuela
Maggie Bowyer
Marguerita Cruz-Urbanc
Mike Baker
Morten Naess
Natalie Murtagh
Nisha Pearson
Prabhjot Kaur Nijjar
Rachael Hird-Smith
Sarah Mills
Saskia Ayre
Savannah Dasilva
Sharon Teji
Sheridan T
Stacey Smith
Stewart Craigon
Susanne Jenssen
Sydney Doberstein Larock
Terrence Conway
Tori Pearmain
Verity Kerr -Morrall
Zoe Almendarez

Thank you for taking the time to read '1-IN-10 Poetry' and supporting Project 514 415. Whether you sought to understand life with endometriosis or have a personal connection to it, I hope that you have discovered solace, validation, knowledge and empathy for people living with endometriosis.

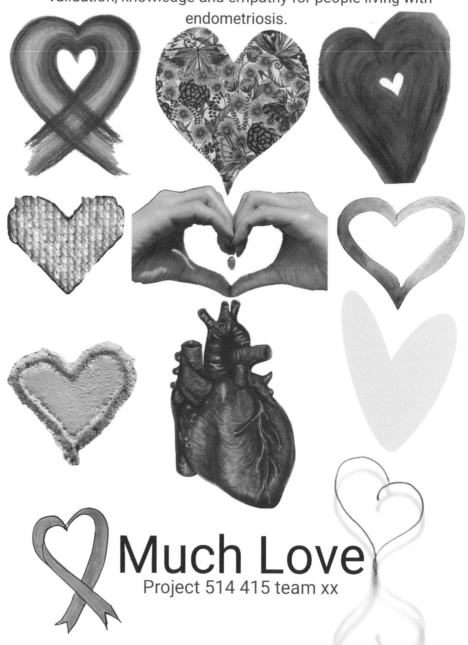

Much Love
Project 514 415 team xx

Author, Founder and Editor

Verity Kerr-Morrall began her career as a dancer and PT; later graduating with a degree in Sports Therapy, and a postgrad in Physiotherapy. Today she is a self-proclaimed creative and the founder of Satriev, using her skillset to encourage empathic learning and empowering health and well-being choices.

CEO of Project 514 415 and Co-Editor

Chelsea Hardesty is an endometriosis advocate and patient, a volunteer representative and research assistant with the Nezhat Family Foundation EndoMarch, a business owner, and founder of Getting the Better of Endometriosis. Chelsea speaks at events, on podcasts, is a published writer, and exhibiting artist.

Chelsea would like to give thanks to her loving husband, mother and children, who have not only supported her with Project 514 415, but with all her endometriosis treatment and advocacy works.

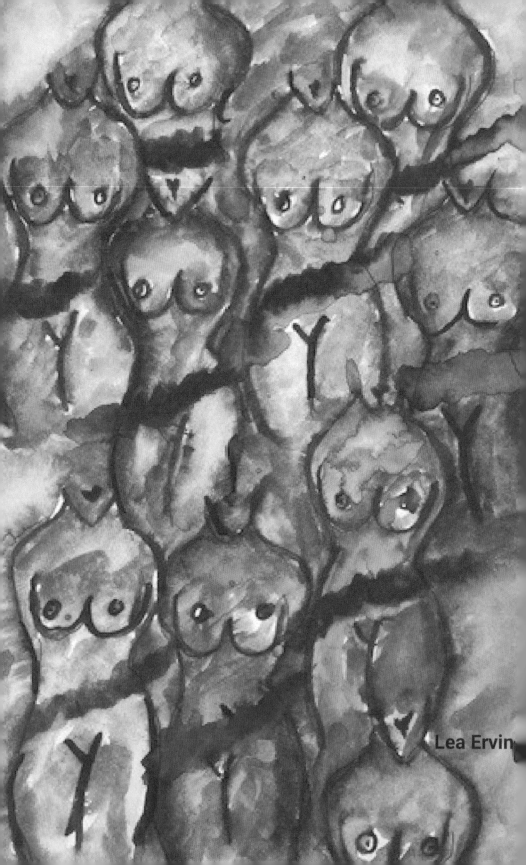

Lea Ervin

Printed in Great Britain
by Amazon

44948094R00137